# The Healing of Trauma during Pregnancy, Birth, and the First Years of Life

**PSYCHOANALYTIC STUDIES:**

**Clinical, Social, and Cultural Contexts**

**Series Editor:** Michael O'Loughlin, Adelphi University

**Mission Statement**

*Psychoanalytic Studies* seeks psychoanalytically informed works addressing the implications of the location of the individual in clinical, social, cultural, historical, and ideological contexts. Innovative theoretical and clinical works within psychoanalytic theory and in fields such as anthropology, education, and history are welcome. Projects addressing conflict, migrations, difference, ideology, subjectivity, memory, psychiatric suffering, physical and symbolic violence, power, and the future of psychoanalysis itself are welcome, as are works illustrating critical and activist applications of clinical work.

**See** https://rowman.com/Action/SERIES/LEX/LEXPS **for a list of advisory board members.**

**Recent Titles in the Series**

*The Healing of Trauma during Pregnancy, Birth, and the First Years of Life: From Dreaming to Being* by Norma Tracey

*The Borderline Culture: Intensity, Jouissance, and Death* by Željka Matijašević

*In Search of Return: Mourning the Disappearances in Kashmir* by Shifa Haq

*Trauma and Repair: Confronting Segregation and Violence in America* by Annie Stopford

*Psychoanalysis as a Subversive Phenomenon: Social Change, Virtue Ethics, and Analytic Theory* by Amber M. Trotter

*A People's History of Psychoanalysis: From Freud to Liberation Psychology* by Daniel José Gaztambide

*Rethinking the Relation between Women and Psychoanalysis: Loss, Mourning, and the Feminine* edited by Hada Soria Escalante

*Lives Interrupted: Psychiatric Narratives of Struggle and Resilience* edited by Michael O'Loughlin, Secil Arac-Orhun, and Montana Queler

# The Healing of Trauma during Pregnancy, Birth, and the First Years of Life

## From Dreaming to Being

Norma Tracey

LEXINGTON BOOKS
*Lanham • Boulder • New York • London*

Published by Lexington Books
An imprint of The Rowman & Littlefield Publishing Group, Inc.
4501 Forbes Boulevard, Suite 200, Lanham, Maryland 20706
www.rowman.com

86-90 Paul Street, London EC2A 4NE



British Library Cataloguing in Publication Information Available

Library of Congress Cataloging-in-Publication Data Available

ISBN 9781666921267 (cloth)
ISBN 9781666921274 (ebook)

*For Jeff Eaton*
*This book is a celebration of some twenty years of his thinking and supporting of my work and that of my colleagues*

# Contents

# Preface

This book focuses on the inner world during pregnancy, birth and the first years of an infant's life. It combines academic insights with sixty years of practitioner experience to provide an in-depth psychoanalytic analysis for identifying and healing trauma during this period. It concerns a woman's internal world as mother as she transverses the processes of maturity to do with pregnancy and birth, focusing on her inner world, her suffering and her recovery from trauma during this period. It applies to the internal world of the father equally. It also focuses on those women and men who have had very damaged early lives, and the method of treating these in adulthood. Particular focus is on the method of treatment, dating from Aboriginal approaches to trauma, and moving beyond present-day concepts to the therapist who makes use of their own emotions to create a rapport with the patient that is totally involved with an "at-oneness" and yet removed enough to remain totally within the structure of the therapeutic treatment of trauma.

Most relevant are the Chapters gleaned from work over the last twenty-five years with young aboriginal woman during pregnancy, birth and early childhood. What is learnt from these years about transgenerational trauma, social suffering, poverty, abandonment, racial discrimination and neglect is balanced by respect for the young mothers extraordinary resilience and wish to get it right for their children. What enveloped me and my thinking during this time was the depth of spirituality in their culture. This oldest living peoples in the world, they have so much to teach us and we have so much to amend in our understanding of their culture, spirituality and their 'present day' needs. I hope this book goes some way towards achieving this.

# Acknowledgments

The two most important people in my professional life were my analyst Ron Brookes, and my supervisor of over thirty years David Buick. My first paper "The Psychic Space in Trauma" was published in the *Journal of Child Psychotherapy* in London in 1991. Frances Tustin on reading it began a correspondence with me. What I had written was how the autistic core in trauma was created by the shattering of the at-oneness created by the internal implosion, leaving a dead space akin to the autism she spoke of in infants. Frances Tustin quoted pages of my work in a manuscript she sent me, which was later published in an abridged form in *Journal of Child Psychotherapy*. Her thinking deeply influenced my work.

I spent many years enjoying the genius of Mike Eigen, who released me from the dangers of parochial analytic rigidity and gave me freedom to grow and think for myself with confidence. He introduced me to Jeff Eaton. Jeff and I spoke daily and later weekly, and for the last fourteen years he was the leader of discussions in our Sydney Psychotherapy Group on our work with Aboriginal mothers in Gunawirra. I have dedicated this book to him for twenty years of unfailing support.

Over the years there are those US analysts who added and supported me, mainly Marilyn Charles, Michael O'Loughlin, Ingo Lambrecht, and Ioannis Sapountzis. Much of my thinking in my clinical work was tested through their thinking and support in forming Gunawirra and our work there. I want to thank them here, particularly Michael O'Loughlin who is male midwife to this book. Thank you to my wonderful professional team at Gunawirra who created that "Camelotian moment" of what could be done to help our Aboriginal sisters in pregnancy, birth and those early years of motherhood.

Just as I was finishing writing this book, I read a wonderful new work by Ofra Eshel. I saw a line of continuity between Eshel's writing and my thinking with Frances Tustin around the catastrophe of premature loss of the illusion of "at-oneness." We are all writing about the same at-oneness, and how its collapse results in trauma of horrendous proportions—a catastrophe.

Although physical birth occurs after ten months, the psychic birth continues at the very base of our personality through every transitional living experience until we die. This book had the profound effect of putting into words and theory what I had long carried out in clinical practice, often not understanding it but going with my intuition.

Judy Eekhoff, a recent friend to my thinking from Klein, Winnicott, Bion, and Eigen has become an enriching, validating source for my work and my thinking. She is my reader, and as such has helped me throughout this book with her thinking about my clinical work. I thank her. I was in weekly discussion throughout the writing of this book in our Dream Group, made up of Jeff Eaton, Marlene Goldsmith, Keri Kohen, and Luca Panseri. I never directly discussed the book in the group, but I did experience them as an underground river that helped me to make sense of what I was trying to think through.

There were midwives without whom this book would not have been born. The first is Michael O'Loughlin, who as editor of this series was directly receptive of my initial submission and a guide throughout. The other is my ever-present and long-suffering editor Eleanor Brasch. I would no sooner get back an edited chapter than new thoughts would fill my mind around it, and I would want to write it again. My final editor was Paul Stirner in London and I thank him for his contribution and his hard work, which shows on every page. I want to thank Loray Daws my colleague who I have known from the days of Mike Eigen's group.

Finally, I want to thank the editors at Rowman and Littlefield, Judith Lakämper who was courteous and helpful throughout and Jasper Mislak who got me to the point of publication with support and advice. I saw them as assistants to the midwives at every point, but it was their work which made this infant a reality.

Thank you Paul Porteous, my son, who helped me throughout. John my husband would have been proud of us.

I hope my writings here does honor to the help and support I have received over sixty-four years of clinical professional life from many others as well as those I have listed here.

# Cover Story

### "THE HEALING PATH"

The white colored hand is the healthy part of an individual's mind. The grey hand is strangling it and holding it back from moving forward along the path of healing. The grey hand is the power of the transgenerational trauma, which becomes like a darkness—an absolute darkness that inhibits happiness and any living emotion. The black hand is grasping the grey hand, and is trying to free the healthy state of mind, but the grey hand forbids this. The white hand is reaching out for its salvation, the yellow circle in the middle. Its salvation is whatever the individual wants it to be, happiness, children raised better than they were, closure of trauma. The different colored paths going towards it are other people's paths to healing.

This painting is by Michael Mondo, a twenty-year-old Aboriginal and the story is his own.

# Introduction

Let me be clear from the outset. Nothing I write about applies only to women or females of any age. My 64 years of professional experience have demonstrated very strongly that the processes I discuss occur equally in men, males of any age. The physic events of moving from oblivion to being, of preconceptive ambivalence, conception, pregnancy, birth and to new life, are a part of the internal processes of the unconscious mind that occur in every living creature from the living to dying, and can occur at all ages. The unconscious does not discriminate from male to female, the unconscious processes are accentuated by true physical events but occur without physical events. It is in this arena of the inner psychic world processes that I write; regardless of age and sex, they continue from oblivion to womb to tomb.

I realized that long before my life focus was on conception, pregnancy and birth, I had a concept relating to the whole spiritual nature of conception, birth, death, regardless of having physical children or not. They were all spiritual mothers and creative in countless ways, as were their male counterparts. There were many aberrations that I became aware of as an adult, but the purpose of creativity was clear. In therapy where the focus is on the unconscious, one is strongly aware of the non-defined separation from male to female. This is not just as part of the protection of the progeny, it is inherent as part of the normal process of being. Do males and females experience psychic pregnancy and birth—they certainly do. Do males and females have post-natal depression—they certainly do. They are grateful and relieved when these processes are accepted and expression of them is encouraged. The demarcation lines between physical and psychic, between male and female, do not exist in the unconscious.

This book focuses on the inner world during pregnancy, birth and the first years of an infant's life. It combines academic insights with sixty years of practitioner experience to provide an in-depth psychoanalytic analysis for identifying and healing trauma during this period. It concerns a woman's internal world as mother as she transverses the processes of maturity to do with pregnancy and birth, focusing on her inner world, her suffering and her recovery from trauma during this period. It applies to the internal world of the father equally. It also focuses on those women and men who have had very damaged early lives, and the method of treating these in adulthood. Particular focus is on the method of treatment, dating from Aboriginal approaches to trauma, and moving beyond present-day concepts to the therapist who makes use of their own emotions to create a rapport with the patient that is totally involved with an "at-oneness" and yet removed enough to remain totally within the structure of the therapeutic treatment of trauma.

Working in the professorial unit of a children's hospital, I began 62 years of clinical work around a woman's developing, intrapsychic transition and growth during pregnancy and first years of their child's life. As a professional social worker and psychoanalytic psychotherapist I have had personal analysis, weekly supervision for over 40 years, many group studies of the literature, and conducted formal research over 30 to 40 years. I have used the clinical work, and the thinking born from this, many times in published papers, books, lectures and public presentations, and now include these with new chapters for publication. Throughout, I use extracts from research interviews and notes from clinical practice to illustrate my themes—in call cases pseudonyms are used and identities are withheld.

How does trauma during pregnancy and the first years of life disturb and distort normal processes at their core? In the last 20 years, I have centered my thinking around clinical work with Aboriginal pregnant women and mothers, using their ancient cultural dreaming and psychoanalytic thinking to further develop ways of treating and healing trauma. My formal research with transgenerational and present trauma gives this book a depth of understanding, but it was the earlier working in hospitals and in neonatal wards and private practice with depressed mothers that helped develop meaningful processes that could be used with my patients, and more recently in the last 15 years in the challenging work with Aboriginal mothers.

The first research was 250 interviews with ordinary suburban parents. Narratives from this study are in Chapter 3 The next research was with parents of premature infants, which comprised over 150 interviews with mothers and fathers of premature infants and a comparable group of mothers and fathers of full-term infants. This was published in a seminal textbook, *Parents of Premature Infants* (Tracy 2000). In the last 20 years the work with six groups of Aboriginal mothers in regional and rural New South Wales was formally researched by Western Sydney University Medical School.

Any professional who works in a psychoanalytic model will have had a personal analysis for the healing of their own traumas; if that healing occurs, they are emotionally available and able to allow it in others. This personal analysis allowed insights that made the challenging work with young pregnant Aboriginal women possible. This demanded a shift in thinking, with people so traumatized that my team were often dealing not with symbols, not with memories, but with the stark reality of terrible living experiences. It required not losing or abandoning psychoanalytic principles, but holding to them firmly enough to dare to move out of the comfort of that thinking and understanding of symbolic processes into a whole new learning experience, with new ways of thinking and approaching the very serious real problems they presented. This was not only for Aboriginal mothers but for other mothers and men I saw that demanded of me a total immersion while keeping my therapeutic stance. What surprised me most was that my "becoming psychotic" with them brought about such health-giving results. My years of studying Freud, Klein, Winnicott, Bion, and Tustin led me to a place they had described so well, a whole new area of at-oneness with the patient.

From a sociological point of view, Australia is a country of many different cultures. These range from the children of Jewish refugees of the Second World War and young Australian soldiers suffering trauma from that war, to present-day migrants suffering still from the problems of the previous generations of Lebanese, Greeks and Italians, to postwar refugees from Europe and more recent migrants from Vietnam and other Asian countries. Working clinically with these diverse cultures created an awareness of the relevance of psychoanalytic work as a powerful way of repairing trauma. Loss of culture for any race means being cut off from their mother country, from their extended family, and from the meaning of their lives and their identity. Finding meaning in their lives here is what recovery from trauma allows.

Finally, a race of First Nations peoples had been cut off from access to aspects of their culture that might have helped them to accommodate and recover from the trauma of invasion. Their at-oneness with their land, people, culture, and spiritual beliefs was shattered by the superimposing of white man's culture. However, in clinical work over 20 years with Aboriginal mothers and infants I developed an awareness of how ancient Aboriginal "Dreaming" opened the door to symbolization, and how 60,000 years ago, people found a resolution and healing of trauma through a process called Dadirri. It was the forerunner of all trauma work today. The Dreaming was also the forerunner of Freudian emphasis on the relevance of our capacity to dream, whether that be daydreaming or sleep dreaming. Aboriginal Dreaming may well be at the roots of psychic existence, and the earliest man's capacity to symbolize, out of which is born the psychic capacity to "think" an experience and so store it for future use. Trauma makes such thinking impossible; recovering from trauma gives purpose and meaning to the experience of living. The hope is that this book opens thinking for the new generation of social workers and psychologists, psychotherapists and psychoanalysts, so that with its publication, a small brick will be put in the edifice of intrapsychic understanding of trauma.

## A MAP OF THIS BOOK

This introduction gives the reason, history, and purpose of this book, including a map through a description and a brief summary of what each chapter brings. Each chapter is informed by my professional work of over 60 years. Throughout, I give particular credence to the Aboriginal concepts that link us to Dadirri and to "the Dreaming." This book is not just about trauma, or even the healing of trauma. This book is also about the spiritual origins of creativity. In the Aboriginal sense, creative does not belong to the individual but to the ecology of earth and its life processes.

Chapter 1 attempts to define psychic trauma? It presents the idea of Dadirri, used by ancient Aboriginals and known as "deep soul listening" and "the Dreaming," which is central to all healing of trauma. It identifies a central autistic core in trauma. The chapter goes on to define the nature of trauma as a psychic wound. Put simply, the events causing trauma cannot be processed; they become thingified and are not able to be converted to symbols, models or abstraction, and so cannot be stored for future use. This chapter seeks to understand the depth of trauma in earliest life not just as a dissociation, but as a total catastrophe leading to psychic deadness. It presents this deadness as an autistic core at the center of trauma. It enunciates the process by which this deadness can be brought to new life through therapy.

Chapter 2 lays the foundation of what occurs in trauma in pregnancy, prematurity, birth and early years of a mother's internal world, defining the psychoanalytic processes during pregnancy. For every human being—male and female and non-binary—there is a continuing dynamic process of pregnancy, rebirth and regrowth in every psychic phase of their lives, from conception to death.. For the woman, it never so profoundly affects her real life as when there is a real pregnancy—a physical baby. Here the psychic and physical processes coalesce. Through the psychic processes of pregnancy, a woman "awakens" as a mother in an emotional sense. Becoming a mother means moving towards a surrender of her infantile passions and desires to meet the needs of her infant; she mediates between a backward pull to passive being and a forward push to active becoming, and she separates from her inner idealized mother to confront the terror of death from her inner destructive one. Hopefully, she survives this to become an alive mother to her infant. In her mind she creates a "womb space" where her internal representation of her pregnancy resides. This is a continuing dynamic. She works with the dialectic between life and death, love and hate, from preconception, through pregnancy, birth, and every life stage. Parallel processes occur in her partner and her infant. It is important that this be known and understood.

In Chapter 3 I study of the effects of trauma during pregnancy. There are marked changes in the psyche's normal functioning created by trauma. This chapter is born out of my many years interviewing pregnant mothers and fathers, and my study of the effects of trauma on dynamics during pregnancy. Case studies and narratives are born out of my 150 interviews with pregnant women and their partners in traumatizing circumstances.

Chapter 4 is a study of psychotherapy with a traumatized pregnant woman who the year before had experienced the death of her first infant on the day it was born. This touches deeply the very core of psychotic "death," where trauma resides.

Chapter 5 is a case study of a hospital team's work with a mother and father who lost one twin in intensive care soon after birth and, in terror, could not acknowledge the life of the other twin still in hospital. How does trauma affect the remembering and storing and processing of an experience? How does trauma affect the capacity to change an experience into an abstraction or a model and store it for further use? How does trauma destroy links? How are these restored?

Chapter 6 illustrates how my work has developed over the years and how my thinking about, and work with, depressed mothers has evolved. It draws on a central theme: the depressed mother, returning to her own infant beginnings through pregnancy and birth, confronts a dead mother–dead infant dyad. Trauma from the mother's own infancy is seen to have created an internal, autistic, deadened, psychic space. It is argued that behind this deadness lies the primeval pain of abandonment and loss. The associated rage, previously repressed but now awakened by her alive infant and its powerful primitive demands, invade the mother's psyche. The internal deadness freezes her alive processes as mother to and Suszie. may experience herself as drowning in something catastrophic.

Chapter 7 is on the psychic reality of becoming a mother. It is about a psychic process; a process through which a woman becomes a mother. In this transition to motherhood, she mediates between a backward pull to passive being, and a forward push to active becoming. She separates from her inner idealized mother to confront the terror of death from her inner destructive one; she wins through to become an alive mother to her infant. This is a continuing dynamic. She works with the dialectic of life and death, love and hate, from preconception, through pregnancy, birth and every life stage. Parallel processes occur in her partner and her infant, and while acknowledging the value of the father and the importance of mother-father interaction, the focus here is on a woman's internal world as mother. The chapter highlights intergenerational gender processes and their effect on motherhood through presenting segments of my therapeutic interactions with four mothers. These portray each mother's dramatic struggle against internal, infantile regressive forces, as she pushes her way out, and awakens to give birth to herself as a mother. I explore how a therapist can facilitate a mother to work through her unresolved conflicts.

In Chapter 8, on the autistic core in trauma, I return to the idea of Dadirri used by ancient Aboriginals and known as "deep soul listening" and explores how "the Dreaming" with Dadirri is central to all healing of trauma. I identify a central autistic core in trauma, which I first published in a paper called "The Psychic Space in Trauma" (Tracey 1991). Frances Tustin responded to this paper in the same journal and was thereafter in communication with me until she died, calling me her "kindred spirit across the ocean." This chapter goes on to define the nature of trauma as a serious psychic wound. The event causing the trauma cannot be processed. It becomes thingified, unable to be converted to symbols or abstraction, and therefore cannot be stored for use. It explains what happens to internal objects in trauma, to knowing and unknowing and the loss of symbolization and identity. It sees psychic death as a direct result of trauma, with the case studies forming an illuminating background to this problem.

Chapter 9 discusses the processes taking place in the movement from oblivion to becoming, as we traverse from nothing to something. How does trauma then take us from something to nothing? How do these processes create, impede or destroy psychic birth? In this earliest of all psychic events, use is made of a particular state of mind, called paradox. It looks at the mother with her infant in the very beginning of her infant's psychic birth as a person, and her psychic birth as the mother to that infant. The mother and infant create a paradigm of what is repeated over and over in therapeutic work with patients. The meaning of how one views one's work with patients is discussed, with case material to identify this vital process. A case discussion highlights the trauma of prematurity.

Chapter 10, on precreative space, is about Aboriginal culture, going back maybe 50,000 years, experiencing the physical place where the young Aboriginal woman was pregnant and gave birth to her baby as sacred ground, always revered by her and her community. That place, the young pregnant suburban Aboriginal woman of today must reclaim, but now, instead of being land, it is the space of her body, mind, and emotions. She needs to reclaim this space from alcohol, drugs, and violence and declare it once more a sacred place for holding life and giving birth—the sacred land of new beginnings—not only for her infants, but for herself and her community.

Chapter 11 draws on my 15 years in a professional team working with traumatized Aboriginal infants and children in their early years of life. This chapter focuses on direct work with traumatized children, where the teacher and the health professional are involved.

Chapter 12 demonstrates the relevance of earliest infancy trauma and its effect through to adulthood. It gives clinical details of the long and intense task of healing, of naming the "un-nameable," of giving voice to a no presence until a presence is there. This chapter begins by thinking about the effects of the patient's trauma on the inner psyche of the therapist, and how the working through between the therapist and patient is central to the outcome.

Chapter 13 gives another case study, further revealing the effects on the patient and the therapist of working through trauma.

Chapter 14 is a brief summation of what is central to this book.

All these chapters are around the central issue of finding meaning. The tragedy of trauma is that it denudes meaning from experience, it destroys meaning, one cannot give it words, one cannot allow life, and one cannot symbolize or store it for the future. All this changes through the transformational work between therapist and patient.

## *Chapter 1*

# Psychic Trauma and Its Healing

### DADIRRI

Before time was conceived, eons ago, Aboriginal people's ancestors knew about trauma. Loved ones died, there were battles in which death or serious injury resulted, breakdowns in relationships occurred; attacks, wounds and death by animals were part of everyday living. They were aware of issues not only of physical survival, but also of a need to heal the psyche. The healing of trauma has since these times been integral to survival on our planet. Here is the earliest story given to us today by Aboriginal people. The person in trouble would go to the leader of their own sex. The leader would call the women or the men to join a circle known simply to us now as Dadirri.

Dadirri is the practice of deep listening. This deep listening is central to all healing of trauma. This deep listening is a creation of the illusion of oneness from womb to birth and through the first year. Therapists in treating trauma use themselves in this earliest process. In cases of personal trauma, social trauma, cultural trauma, world trauma created by wars, disease, fire, flood, famine, present-day practitioners seek a way of healing trauma. In doing so, Dadirri offers a basic paradigm of "deep listening" as central to all treatment of trauma. The Dadirri process mirrors much of the intrapsychic action of a mother with her infant; to receive pain, to hold it, to process it, to give it back in a tolerable form. This is central to all psychic healing. My thoughts are that it is in this earliest breakdown of "at-oneness" with the mother, the infant ego is catastrophically shattered. A kind of psychic deadness results. Through therapy, life can not just be restored but in fact may be experienced for the first time.

This book is in the area of psychological birth and psychological catastrophe. I want to add Aboriginal Dreaming as an important part of the healing—this creates illusion and symbols that give inner meaning to the world around us; it is crucial to the healing of trauma. Trauma concretizes the experience so it cannot be thought of or imagined. It is a death to dreaming. The healing of trauma allows thinking and symbolization of the experience, so it is no longer the concreted "thing in itself," but has an internal symbolization of the experience that creates of it a model and an abstraction for future use. Therefore, this book is predicated on two significant gifts from ancient Aboriginal peoples: the concept of Dadirri and the concept of the Dreaming. Ancient ancestral dreaming was the beginning of how we as humans imbued our external world and events with meaning from our inner world; we create boundaries for this meaning; we create symbols for it.

## Central to the Healing of Trauma Is Deep Soul Listening Known as Dadirri

In Dadirri, the person experiencing trauma is invited to speak, and through this speech communicates their pain; the group listens, but it is listening of a special kind, a deep soul listening, a hearing in the depth of one's being. It is the capacity of the group to experience with the traumatized person the sense of at-oneness. Empathy of a very special kind allows this hearing, making intolerable pain, tolerable; the unthinkable, able to be thought about. Empathy breaks through the concreted psychic deadness, allowing the pain to be felt and shared, so the experience can be tolerated and digested. This process is identical to a mother's earliest interactions with her baby. A mother listens. In the depth of her being, she hears the infant's cries, a response is awakened, because they are as one. Early after birth her response is immediate, as infant life depends on it, not just physically but psychically. Later, an internal living image of a breast that feeds and a mother that comforts are in the mind of the infant (Bion 1977). This internal imaging of a satisfying experience holds the infant until the mother comes. This is the "dreaming." In the beginning, the mind cannot hold these thoughts, so a real presence is needed—a real mother to hold the infant. In the absence of the mother the infant tries to hold itself by movement, by cries for help that carry hope of being heard, and sometimes if that help does not come, Bowlby gives us an image of the whole system closing down and the infant giving up (Bowlby 1969). Bion (1977), Tustin (1981) and Eigen (2004a) define this as the catastrophe ending in psychic death. Recovery is the same internal action as Dadirri, and the processes of emotional interaction as expressed by Bion, Tustin and Eigen are taking place. But here, it is the group that holds the person's pain, that empathizes with the pain and by that empathy makes it bearable. All the senses are involved, not just hearing, but seeing the pain in the other person's body and actions and experiencing that pain with them. These groups went on and on, sometimes for hours, until the person signaled that he could now tolerate his pain and, by digesting it, allow it to enter his psyche to become part of his inner experience (Bion 1977). Recovery in the therapeutic process requires a space like Dadirri where suffering the suffering in the suffering can occur, where the "words to say it" can be found, where freedom of speech is allowed, where careful silence monitors and negotiates the amount and timing of how much the person in trauma can tolerate (Joseph 1981). The central psychosis of terror and death is neutralized; the paradox of that terror of being and of that terror of being annihilated is dispelled by the psychic holding. The mother does that; the healing circle of Dadirri does that; the good-enough therapist in any psychoanalytically informed therapy does that. Like Dadirri, like early motherhood, the therapeutic encounter liberates the capacity to dream, giving a renewed womb where new fetal symbolism can occur.

## THE AUTISTIC CORE IN TRAUMA

Understanding trauma has been for me a long journey of many years of working in neonatal intensive care, resulting in my paper, "The Psychic Space in Trauma" (1991), which speaks to a deadened central autistic area resulting from trauma. From this was born my work with Frances Tustin (1994). Later, Tustin's work looking at the catastrophe of rupturing the psychic at-oneness in early infancy, first published in 1981, became the center of all my work. It formed the basis of my research over four years into the trauma suffered by parents of premature infants (Tracey 2000). Jeff Eaton and I shared much of our thinking, further developing ideas around trauma which I shared when I wrote *Precreative Space* (2009). The central place of "at-oneness" was meaningfully developed through Ofra Eshel's book, *The Emergence of Analytic Oneness* (2019), which arrived as I was finishing this book. I found myself so in tune with her thinking about the relevance of the shattering of the unconscious illusion of "at-oneness." It added so much to my understanding of the way meaning is stripped away because of trauma, and how psychotic autistic states can result. At the same time, the publication of Judy Eekhoff's book, *Trauma and Primitive Mental States* (2019), has taken us to the center of the catastrophe of trauma. In her work with adults who as newborn babies were temporarily separated from their mothers for medical reasons, she defines the autistic effects that this rupture at birth creates through to adulthood. "Thingifying" occurs in trauma that is unresolved so that the experience remains the thing in itself. This has a physical equivalent, as in severe trauma when the amygdala closes down from the hippocampus, so no processing of the experience can occur. It remains the experience as a nightmare that cannot be dreamt. Her work adds to the meaning of somatic events resulting from trauma.

> Trauma is a psychic wound, caused by a violent intrusion. An excess of psychic pain floods the ego. Projective identification fails as a container. The psychic pain becomes unbearable and there is fear of fragmentation and death. Internal objects are destroyed, omnipotence takes their place, so there is no mourning. There is unthinkable fear, so there is no thinking, and hence no symbolization. The experience of negative feelings is greater than that of positive ones, causing archaic denial and regression to primary processing, instead of repression and secondary processing. What is left is a non-living space, where knowing would be it if could be known, where thought would be it if could be thought. This space has an autistic, deadening quality I have called the autistic core, which is demonstrably similar to that described in autistic children by Tustin. (Tracey 1991, 29)

Laplanche and Pontalis (1973, 466) write that in a psychic trauma there are three implicit ideas: "The idea of violent shock, the idea of a wound, and the idea of consequences affecting the organization." Freud (1963, 275) speaking of trauma, says: "We apply it to an experience which within a short period of time presents the mind with an increase of stimulus too powerful to be dealt with, or worked off in the normal manner." Bion (1977) says there is a violent explosion, accompanied by immense psychotic fear or panic, expressed by a sudden total silence to get away from the devastation. Perhaps the theorist most helpful in describing trauma resulting from loss is Bowlby (1969), who writes of a state of protest, which if unmet brings despair and psychic detachment. This detachment is the autistic deadened space. Trauma in medicine means wound. In the Greek language, "wound" means "pierce."

Freud's comments in "Draft A" of the Fleiss Papers seem to be a metaphor for what we might surmise is happening. "It is like a 'wound,' an 'internal haemorrhage, a hole in the psychic sphere'" (Freud 1966, 177–78). According to Pontalis (1981, 196), "an excess of excitation hinders and binds activity, at the level of primary process." Klein (1946) wrote of an early mechanism of defense called projective identification. In her view, the infant defends his ego from intolerable anxiety by splitting off and projecting unwanted feelings and impulses into his mother. This binds the stimulus and relieves him. When the mother fails emotionally to do this, Bick (1968) says a psychic hole is made like a wound in his emotional skin and the infant fears his emotions will pour through this hole. There is a terror of himself pouring through it and suffering annihilation. In the absence of a holding mother. the child is left to attempt to hold his own stimulus and it is suggested his failure to do so sends him hurtling back to the black hole of primary repression (Kingston and Cohen 1986). Lewis (1983, 209) describes it thus: "A black hole is a star with an extraordinary dense mass whose gravitational pull is so powerful that no energy can escape from it, so that it appears to us as a nothing, a black hole in space."

## Breakdown

This "autistic cut-out" psychic space is a normal primitive defense that works to protect the person from over stimulus. "We are born with a safety valve through which we become numb to pain, inured to meanings that are unmanageable. This safety valve enables us to survive the unsurvivable" (Charles 2014, 25). Too much emotion is itself experienced as traumatic and the child shuts down. Trauma thus not only cuts us off from what is happening in the moment, but also from the self-regulatory capacities that might help us cope (Charles 2014, 25). That very capacity for disassociation, to distance from self and experience to survive the moment, impedes integration and repair and a mastery of an experience that gives self-esteem. It is even more serious, for trauma disrupts narrative coherence and disjunctive behavior in the parents, avoiding their own unresolved trauma, making them unavailable at the very moment the child most needs them. What is most important following on from Charles's thinking is how much the trauma of the parents, with lots of culture, of family, of spirituality, of the meaning of living, is now being passed on to their children, and breakdown is ensuing from this. In extreme cases such as trauma in early infancy, or childhood, or in severe adult trauma, the defense becomes concretized, a psychotic core. Emotion is unable to be experienced, pain is unable to be suffered, meaning is lost and "thingifying" or concretization causes loss of internal reverie and empathy. Perhaps this is what may have happened to Aboriginal people when they were cut off from their culture, community, and earth place: meaning became lost for them. Far more seriously, what they also lost was their ancient ritualistic or customary ways of dealing with trauma. At the other extreme, the autistic defense does not hold and "breakdown" results for some. Chaos, envy, and rage overflow, with ensuing primitive enactment, which may include criminality. Many Aboriginal people now have the problem of severe addiction, which may initially be an effort to quell the nightmare of such mad emotions enacted as violence, rape, murder or suicide. In such cases they have no internal holding boundaries to protect themselves or others from the primitive overflow.

## Ego Processes are Deadened in Trauma

Freud (1957a), Klein (1946) and Bion (1977) are aware of the regression caused by trauma. The logic of the unconscious takes over with some bizarre results. The unconscious mind makes up how it wishes things to be and denies what it does not want to know. Omnipotence of thought is a defense against extreme psychic pain. Marion Milner (1987) describes omnipotence and omniscience of thought as a protection against impotence and lack of capacity to control. Guilt is born out of a belief in the power to direct and cause. The traumatized person experiences himself as having killed his internal objects. That space is where the conscious mind would be active and where symbolization is now deadened. But in trauma the unconscious rules—it does not have time, it does not have space, it displaces one event with another as if all events are the same. Freud described these functions of the unconscious in 1900 in *The Interpretation of Dreams* (see Freud 1995). For Matte-Blanco (1986), the traumatized person has no time, has no inner and outer, no symbolism, is concretized, has no expression or feeling of emotion, and clings to facts of the experience rather than the emotion of that experience. Trauma loses processing into thoughts. This means the events are repressed as the experience itself.

## The Loss of Symbolism

In trauma there is a loss of capacity to symbolize. I will explain this by using Bion's (1977) constructs concerning "thinking." From birth there are inborn preconceptions; take, for example, the breast, there can be a preconception of a breast that satisfies or a breast that does not satisfy. Once there is an actual event of a satisfactory breast, the emotion linked to the experience at the breast combines with the preconception. If the meeting of a preconception and an event is positive, emotional affect is alive; the experience is kept and stored, and a model is abstracted for future reference. There is a living dynamic of "getting to know." A metaphor of what might go on is available, so symbolization is possible. There can be a future without fear of needing to get to know again and again. What then, when the meeting of a preconception and the real event causes a conception of something truly terrible? What when the preconception of an alive and growing baby becomes a dead baby? The emotional experience becomes unbearable. The area is deadened. Instead of storage in a safe container, it is evacuated. Such an experience is concretized; it has no emotional effect, it can only be stored as the thing in itself, not as a model for future use (Tracey 1991).

## Archaic Denial in Trauma

In trauma it is the psychic action of archaic denial rather than repression that causes the dead or autistic space. How does this come about? I use once more a basic paradigm—the breast. From the first feed, an image of a satisfying breast is stored. "This internal breast imago—a memory image of a past gratifier—serves as a substitute object, and like the discharge of effect which accompanies it, tides the baby over a time of distress" (de Monchaux 1962, 311). The timing and the dosage of frustration before relief allow a thought of something gratifying to be kept. There is not only an idea of a positive hallucination when there is an absence, but the reality of an absence. If absence can be tolerated, hallucination of a bad breast can occur and the positive and negative hallucinations can neutralize each other and be canceled out. In this neutralizing action the affect is repressed and the result is thought. In trauma the affect is denied, and the result is no thought. When there is no thought (secondary processing), there is a regression to hallucinatory images (primary processing). When this happens, the negative persecutory hallucination is so powerful it fragments the positive hallucination. The fragments are de-cathected because they are no longer the object desired but fragments. The objects are destroyed, a dead space ensues and omnipotence takes over. What is avoided and hated is ignored and denied any existence. Denial of truth, not repression allowing thought, occurs. The dead or autistic space is where truth would reside if truth could be known and hence thought (Tracey 1991).

## Thingifying

In trauma meaning is lost. The event is frozen in the traumatized person's psyche; they cannot dream or imagine it. There is an intensely destructive space where that which is created is turned into a nothing. The meaning of what the person gives to something is annihilated, and indeed the person is thingified, that is made concrete, tangible. In a healthy resolution, the end result is an interplay between being and not being, meaning and no meaning, something and nothing. These spaces are so opposite, one is a good space in which one can become, and its opposite is a concept of a space where becoming ought to be but is not. From the research interviews conducted for *Parents of Premature Infants* (Tracey 2000), revelation in every parent interview gave credence to how in trauma the experience is concrete, factual, and devoid of affect. This is one mother's narrative:

> After the operation they took me straight back to intensive care, and they expected me to be on the ventilation machine for three weeks. I was lucky that I recovered so quickly and was only on it for two days. For the first couple of days I was pretty much out of it, and unconscious for about the first 36 hours. I really didn't wake up until Saturday morning; that's when they removed the ventilation and feeding tube. On Saturday they wheeled me over the road to the main hospital so that I could see my baby for the first time in the nursery. I was then moved to Brighton 10 E, and this is where I am now. (Tracey 2000, 65)

These are my contemporaneous notes on this testimony:

> Debbie is shaky and breathless as she talks and her whole body is tremulous. I experienced Debbie as unemotional, cut off and dull. It seems paradoxical that she seems deadened but her whole body is shaking and she has difficulty

> breathing, yet it is as if she is reporting on someone else. I thought in her traumatized mind, language has no emotional meaning for her; [research discussants] saw this as a fragmented state, holding the facts together to create a full rather than a fragmented skin on the wound created by trauma. (Tracey 2000, 65)

## Catastrophe and Death

In *Psychic Deadness* (2004a, 60) Eigen notes that "throughout his writings, Bion explores the sense of catastrophic formlessness and its role in creativeness and psychosis." This leads to a "temptation to fill in, to thingify, or otherwise to nullify no-thing is ubiquitous. . . . [It creates] a certain rigidity, tied to defective or embryonic apparatus" (Eigen 2004a, 45). Eigen adds that an analytic interpretation may kill or support the growth of experience, including the experience of violation. He writes of the relevance of allowing the meaningless to exist. "To the extent that the analyst falls victim to his goodwill and soothes meaninglessness away, he may be hated for joining a lie" (Eigen 2004a, 60).

Psychotics cannot stay in the catastrophe, but because they cannot remain in it they cannot leave it. For the psychotic the catastrophe continues underneath, for it has not been dealt with. The psychotic, having destroyed the potential of birth and new life, is stuck in the deadness. The illness of the psychotic is not the hallucination but the fact of being cut off from the empathy with it. In the preface to *The Psychotic Core*, Eigen (2004b, vii) writes, "Bion's work, like Winnicott's, focuses on the sense of catastrophe that underlies psychotic experience. Even the term *annihilation anxiety* does not do justice to the nameless dread that pervades psychosis. The very namelessness of the dreaded catastrophe stamps the experience with an unknown and perhaps unknowable factor." In psychosis, the transmuting of beta elements into food for thought runs amok. These become "failed thoughts" instead of "reborn thoughts." Rather than giving meaning to the emotions, the psychotic destroys the meaning in them. The psychotic is continually in the catastrophe, and yet is so split off as to seem totally out of it (Eigen 2004a). The birth of self "evolves" and "dissolves" around a sense of catastrophe to use the thinking of Eigen and Bion. To reach the central core of becoming we need first to be in the nothing. This requires an internal tolerance born out of faith, a faith that holds regardless, a faith that means groping in the dark, never finding truth, but believing in it always. Donald Winnicott took the view that you cannot consider the development of the child without taking into account its external environment, particularly in the varying interactions with parent figures. Winnicott saw the ego as arising out of primitive threats to existence and developing a "continuity of being," as afforded by the good-enough mother. "The first ego organization comes from the experience of threats of annihilation which do not lead to annihilation and from which, repeatedly, there is recovery" (Winnicott 1984b, 304).

> With "the care that it receives from its mother" each infant is able to have a personal existence, and so begins to build up what might be called *a continuity of being*. On the basis of this continuity of being, the inherit potential gradually develops into an individual infant. If maternal care is not good enough then the infant does not really come into existence, since there is no continuity of being; instead, the personality becomes built on the basis of reactions to environmental impingement. (Winnicott 1960, 595)

Initially, the carer's role is to support the illusion of a fused, undifferentiated unity. The carer then gradually and carefully allows disillusionment where the child realizes its (and its carer's) individuality. This separation happens through play and the use of a transition object (Winnicott 1960).

## The Premature Rupture of the At-oneness

Bion (1977) saw projective identification not as a defense but as a mode of communication, by which the infant lets his mother know what he is feeling. Thus, the feeling, known, shared, and divested of its fear by the containing mother, is made tolerable and can be kept. When the mother is absent or emotionally not able to hold his projection, it "results in the introjection of an object that is hostile to understanding, together with the frightened part of himself. Because it cannot elicit a response it is divested of meaning, this is then experienced as a 'nameless dread'" (Harris 2011, 141). Feelings of despair evoke a need for denial, and denial means no access to emotional content and hence no processing. Eshel (2019) connects explicitly the unknown and unknowable emotional reality—"O"—with unthinkable breakdown (Winnicott) and catastrophe (Bion). Bion and later Tustin considered the detail of how the infant transitions from undifferentiated unity to independence and a realization of the mother as a separate person. The psychological birth is so much slower and occupies the first months of life. The infant resides in the womb of the mother's mind. In every trauma, and central to all that I write in this book, is the idea of catastrophe relating to breakdown in psychological birth, created by the premature rupture of the at-oneness. For this I am grateful to Frances Tustin who wrote to me many times about premature or mismanaged psychological birth as the cause of traumatic catastrophic breakdown resulting in psychotic states. Bion (1977) notes that the mother's capacity for empathic reflexion "reverie" shows how the infant is psychologically in the mind of the mother, in the womb of her mind. To fall out of the mind prematurely is catastrophic. Eshel (2019, 149) writes that this is not in the oedipal world, but rather in the world of Pentheus, Euripides's most tragic hero—a world dominated by a mixture of a mother's madness, devourment, destruction, and rituals of desire.

## COUNTERTRANSFERENCE: THE THERAPIST TREATING TRAUMA

For many of my years of clinical practice, going to "sleep," being blocked from any advance or any experience, being in a numbed state, was extremely costly to me as therapist. Only in understanding the relevance of the at-oneness and the results of psychic health made it worthwhile. Trauma according to Ofra Eshel (2019) has created an "autotomous" massive splitting defense in the service of psychic survival within a violent and deeply traumatic early childhood. Eshel emphasizes the importance of the analyst's abiding "presencing" and "withnessing" or interconnectedness with the traumatized perverse patient, which gradually creates a new, alternative experiential-emotional reality within the patient's alienated world. One needs to be highly respectful of the defenses, for hidden under them is an "extreme collapse into profound devastation, emptiness, psychic death, and violent, suicidal despair" (Eshel 2019, 231). Working in analysis within this collapse enables the deep reason for the patient's breakdown in early life to unfold. And, most importantly, it engenders the crucial possibility that had never been experienced before, of reliving the patient's unbearable breakdown and deadness—this time the patient with analyst t(w)ogether—and experientially coming through it differently. Eshel offers a clinically based framework through which adult survivors of early childhood trauma can re-engage with painful past events to create meaningful futures for themselves. She highlights the use of the body and the mind in working with these early unmentalized and unrepresented states, illustrating the value of finding language that embodies emotions, and working in the here and now of transference and countertransference.

Eshel's writing explores a fundamental dimension of analytic work created by the analyst/therapist's "presencing" (being there) within the patient's experiential world and the grip of the analytic process, and the ensuing deep patient-analyst interconnectedness or "withnessing" that may grow into at-onement with the patient's innermost emotional reality of unthinkable breakdown and catastrophic psychic trauma. This dimension, with its profound ontological implications, engenders markedly new possibilities for extending the reach of psychoanalytic treatment to more disturbed patients and more difficult treatment situations. It goes beyond contemporary analytic notions of intersubjectivity and witnessing to more radical patient-analyst deep-level analytic oneness.

I think that understanding this psychic action has profound implications for therapy. There are specific, definable therapeutic techniques by which this dead inner space may be restored to a psychic living experience. In therapy, this deadened area becomes a space where agony previously avoided is tolerated, despair held, psychic pain of loss suffered and fear contained. Awareness of dosage and timing is all too relevant. Interpretation that focuses on love and hate or good and evil in the patient can be persecutory. Analytic therapy focuses on archaic denial, and the fear, sometimes terror, of "knowing." Psychic holding is the primary therapist-patient interaction. If this internal holding is no longer adequate because of the intensity of the trauma, external holding is necessary for its resolution.

## Biological Changes in Trauma

In his book *The Body Keeps the Score* (2014), Bessel Van Der Kolk highlights that traumatic stress is at the root of neuroscience. What is currently known is that exposure to trauma leads to a cascade of biological changes and stress responses. These biological alterations are highly associated with post-traumatic stress disorder (PTSD), other mental illnesses and substance use disorders.

> Traumatized people chronically feel unsafe inside their bodies: The past is alive in the form of gnawing interior discomfort. Their bodies are constantly bombarded by visceral warning signs, and, in an attempt to control these processes, they often become expert at ignoring their gut feelings and in numbing awareness of what is played out inside. They learn to hide from their selves." (Van der Kolk 2014, 97)

Physiological responses include changes in limbic system functioning; fluctuations in hypothalamic–pituitary–adrenal axis activity with variable cortisol levels; and neurotransmitter-related dysregulation of arousal and endogenous opioid systems.

Traumatic stress is also associated with functional and chemical changes in the emotional part of the brain—the limbic area and brain stem. Knowing the functions of the amygdala, hippocampus, and prefrontal cortex as the primary stress responders in the brain can provide a new therapeutic direction for PTSD management. The hyperactive status of the amygdala triggers the release of stress hormones (Badura-Brack et al. 2018) and impairs the functioning of the hippocampus, causing traumatic memories to remain vivid. In addition, the deactivation of the prefrontal cortex function and the failure to maintain a balanced stress hormone system, causes panic, agitation, and hypervigilance responses in PTSD patients. This hyperactive aroused emotional status can be evidenced by hyperactive brain waves over the fear center of the brain's right temporal lobe, with suppression of electric activity over the frontal area. At the point when one feels undermined, the body discharges chemicals called cortisol and adrenaline. This is the body's programmatic method of getting ready to react to peril.

This can have a range of impacts:

- Freeze—feeling deadened or incapable to move
- Flop—doing what is advised without having the option to dissent
- Battle—battling or dissenting
- Flight—covering up or moving ceaselessly
- Grovel—attempting to satisfy the somebody who hurts the subject

Studies have shown that pressure signs can proceed long after the emotional trauma is finished. This may influence the psyche and body, including thinking, feeling and carrying on. Hyperarousal is a consequence of biological changes initiated by trauma. Although it serves as a means of self-protection after trauma, it can be detrimental. Hyperarousal can interfere with an individual's ability to take the necessary time to assess and appropriately respond to a specific input, and it can produce overreactions to situations perceived as dangerous when, in fact, the circumstances are safe (van de Kolk 2014, 145).

## INTERGENERATIONAL TRAUMA

There is a concern in this book with transgenerational trauma. Davoine and Gaudillière (2004) have worked extensively with individuals for whom unresolved intergenerational trauma has manifested in disrupted life narratives and psychotic symptoms. These authors highlight ways in which trauma speaks across generations in encoded form, speaking whatever has become unspeakable within the family. Psychotic symptoms often capture in concrete terms the metaphors and family myths affecting family members without being overtly recognized. Unacknowledged and unresolved trauma remains free to haunt, distort and undermine development. Judith Atkinson (2002) writes of trauma trails; the disasters of colonization that brought disorder and disharmony. To this day, many Aboriginal families "reflect the pain that came with the disasters of the colonial proceeds: large-scale epidemics; massacres; removal of children through a whole generation; physical and cultural genocide" (Atkinson 2002, 13). Worst of all, Atkinson notes, was the trauma resulting from the destruction of relationships between people and their land and between themselves.

*Chapter 2*

# Inner World Processes During Pregnancy

## INTRODUCTION

There is, for each human being, a continuing dynamic process of pregnancy, rebirth, and regrowth in every psychic phase of life from conception to death. For the woman, it never so profoundly affects her real life as when there is a real pregnancy—a physical baby. Here the psychic and physical processes coalesce. Through the psychic processes of pregnancy, a woman "awakens" as a mother in an emotional as well as a physical sense. Becoming a mother means moving towards a surrender of her infantile passions and desires to meet the needs of her infant; she mediates between a backward pull to passive being, and a forward push to active becoming. Psychically she separates from her idealized inner mother to confront the terror of death from a destructive inner one; hopefully, she survives this to become an alive mother to her infant. She creates a "womb space" in her mind, where her internal representation of her pregnancy resides. This is a continuing dynamic. She works with the dialectic of life and death, love and hate, from preconception, through pregnancy, birth, and every life stage. Parallel processes occur in her partner and her infant. The concepts and processes discussed in this chapter are initially derived from years of study of Bion, Klein, and the Middle School of Object Relations and, more recently, the works of Eigen, Shore, Stern, Eaton, Eshel, and Judy Eekhoff.

## WHAT IS INNER WORLD FANTASY?

The inner world is the place where instincts and experiences of parents and others meet in the form of present living internal representations. Jung (1969) particularly emphasizes that some of these internal representations are universal; some we are born with, inherited from our parents; all are affected by our life experiences and our capacity to process or think, symbolize and retain internal models or representations of life experiences. This chapter is concerned with how an experience is "thought about" and then stored to become part of our internal world. In this internal world, living experiences live a life of their own, with laws quite different from those of the conscious mind, such as there is no distinction between persons; one present person can be experienced as another person in one's history without difference or distinction. This forms the basis of all transference. The inner world has no distinction of time. This is why events of twenty years ago can be experienced as happening right now. There is no capacity to discriminate between the outside and the inside world, which means there is no distinction between inner and outer boundaries or space. This accounts for one believing one's inner world to be real. Psychotic individuals particularly inhabit this space. In this unconscious area, opposites are fused, such as life and death, love and hate, without differentiation or discrimination (Matte-Blanco 1959; Rayner 1981). During pregnancy, the mother leaves the external world and turns toward her inner world, her fetal infant, and her inner psychic infant. In this change, emotions from her inner world are exposed, producing a degree of chaos, and her normal ego functions are therefore lessened. Such a move binds the mother with her infant at the most primitive level. However, such intensity and exposure of emotions creates problems as old conflicts are reactivated, and the pregnant woman is sensitive and vulnerable and in a kind of "madness" as she reaches the birth of herself as a mother and the birth of her infant. It is obvious that an area of the mind that cannot, by itself, discriminate between "alive" and "dead" is chaotic. To give it meaning, "emotional thinking" or processing has to take place. It is out of this processing or emotional thinking that a woman gathers the fragments of herself and finds a new identity that includes motherhood.

How do we process? The mind cannot hold opposites such as life and death or love and hate in the same thought. Rather than fragment or go "mad" by trying to hold these opposites, the mind splits and projects. "Good" may go to one person, "bad" to another (Klein 1946). It is the bringing together of these opposites in a way that is tolerable, rather than fused or split, that gives resolution to an ongoing dynamic. This is where the action of therapy occurs. We process by finding a way in which we can bring the opposites in our inner mind to a meeting place. By doing this, we create a neutral, mediating working area of the mind; love and hate, and life and death sit at the same table as it were to mediate. Hallucinatory primary passions and emotions are surrendered for an emotional compromise of opposites. In such a neutral territory, symbolization and models, conceptualizing and abstracting of our experiences can take place and with these processes, experiences can be mentally and emotionally stored for future use (Bion 1962). It is the acknowledging, identifying and interpreting of the dynamic that makes a psychodynamic psychotherapist. Allowing the movement and free flow of the dynamic is central to our work. Finding the neutral space where thought can occur, where opposites can be tolerated, where symbols, models, and concepts can be born is central to a person's psychic structure.

The three main stages in a woman's life where she experiences deep emotional and physical changes are the onset of puberty, pregnancy, and menopause. In each of these is a maturational crisis marked by chaos. This chaos is a result of the surrender of the old order, giving place to the new. Pregnancy is a time of change, a *maturational crisis*. Several authorities, such as Benedek (1952), have recognized pregnancy as a normal transitional crisis. Bibring (1959), Bibring et al. (1961), and Deutsch (1945) have stressed the profound, sensitive emotional equilibrium of the pregnant woman and her vulnerability to psychological disturbances. A birth involves widespread emotional upheaval; a reappraisal and redefinition of identity occur. These emotions are seen as temporary signs of that change. Pregnancy, therefore, involves profound endocrine and somatic and psychological changes.

The crisis of pregnancy is a normal occurrence, a part of growth that proceeds motherhood. In pregnancy, a woman is born again as a mother. There is for her an awakening of her relationship with her own mother. As with any crisis, there is a renewal of the unresolved conflicts and a chance to resolve them. One is never free of the dynamic of the oedipal phase. In pregnancy, rivalry with the mother is heightened. There is anger toward the mother for making her a girl or gratitude with the mother for her womanhood. There is fear of the mother taking the baby in vengeful reprisal for her anger at the mother, and a fear of not having the mother's love and support. The conscious mind is weakened during pregnancy, the unconscious mind is strengthened. There is conflict in being identified with the mother she had and the mother she wishes she to be. The basic oedipal triangle, with its fantasized sexuality, is revived and repeated—the father-to-be now must share his wife with his child, the wife now has to share the child with the father, and the father with the child, and both parents give up being the only child of the other. From the beginning, a little girl is in conflict with her mother yet identifies with her. Fear is the first conflict. As she gets older, a little girl is rivalrous with her mother for her father. She hates her mother's achievement of sexuality with the father. She thinks the mother in return hates her and wants to destroy her. She also loves her mother and wants to be identified with her. There is guilt. This guilt remains into adolescence. The effort to relieve this and overcome it accounts for the emotional problems of maturation, anorexia nervosa, and bulimia, which are efforts to atone to the mother by never becoming the woman. They may be a defense against sexuality and hence protection against rivalry with the mother, by sexual acting out. This might be by abortion, damaging her own products of creativity to atone for wanting to be like mother.

Listening to a pregnant woman, you will hear how she experiences her internal mother. Hopefully for many the loving feelings will triumph over the negative ones, a space to think will result, and there will be a center from which to grow. If the negative feelings are stronger than the positive ones, no resolution and no thinking space are born. She may have infantile phantasies about herself as the fetus in her mother's body, reawakening intensely ambivalent feelings at a most primitive level. At a more adult level, one of the most satisfying emotions of pregnancy is the identification with an omnipotent, fertile, life-giving mother. She experiences herself as maturing to become a mother in her own right, a physiologically mature woman, impregnated by her sexual partner, powerful enough to create life within herself and hold it.

For many pregnant women, some past external trauma may distort their internal maternal image; a mother has died in childhood; a mother has died during her pregnancy; years of hatred have been nursed from childhood and never acknowledged or resolved; a vulnerable, depressed woman may feel even more depressed in taking over her mother's role and so letting go of her, because pregnancy is the final letting go. When anything goes wrong with the pregnancy, she may experience this as a punishment for her sins.

## SEX AND PREGNANCY

The successful achievement of a feminine sexual gender identity can be strengthened by the proof and confirmation of pregnancy.

> For the primigravida, pregnancy offers proof of a gender identity and the visible manifestation to the outside world that she has had a sexual relationship. Physiologically it is the confirmation that she has a sexually mature body capable of reproduction, but this does not necessarily imply that she has an equally emotionally mature ego, capable of undertaking the responsibilities and demands of parenthood. One of the intrapsychic tasks the young pregnant woman must accomplish involves the internal acceptance of what may be termed the representation of her sexual partner, both physically and mentally. (Deutsch 1945, 143)

## Autonomy in Pregnancy

An embryo is in an amniotic sac in a mother's womb. The fetus has its own internal space. There is a special autonomous space in which the mother and baby reside. The father is the protector of this space. At birth it is "in the womb of the mother's mind" (Tustin 1981, 183). It is in her mind because she thinks about and for it. It is her capacity for reflecting on the fetus's needs that keeps it psychically safe and held. By holding the fetus in her mind, she protects it with her psychic skin until it gets a skin of its own. Intrusion on this is threatening. It destroys both the fetus and her safe place in her mind. There is a line to do with mother-infant autonomy, which is particularly precious for the woman, pregnant with herself as a newborn mother. Intrusion into this vulnerable womb-mind space can cause psychic distress as an intrusion on the fetus can cause physical distress.

When another enters the circle of the mother and her pregnancy, their space is violated, and there is competition with the mother for the baby. One sees this most vividly with a premature infant in a hospital ward, where the place is public; the holder is a humidicrib, the feeder is through tubes. There is medication and the caretaker is not the mother but a ward team. She may well experience them as persecutors and herself as a failure. Equally, and even more so in pregnancy, anything that goes wrong is viewed by her as a failure on her part to be a good caretaker, a good giver. The traumatized woman of this period requires a listening that holds, acts as a shock absorber, and is careful not to judge because she already has a harsh internal mother at war with her.

In a talk he gave at the New South Wales Institute of Psychotherapy in 1988, Professor Berry Brazelton reported:

> We started looking at normal parents, prior to the birth of their babies. We chose five families. We interviewed the mother once a week for the last four months, and father once a month in psychoanalytic interviews. We observed the newborn at birth. They exposed themselves in these interviews with dreams and phantasies that were so disturbing and so disturbed looking, that when we made a prediction from these, they all looked as though they would be psychotic parents. When they had their babies, all this madness and pathology began to shape up as a normal process. We began to realise this turmoil was serving a purpose by dredging up all the alarm reactions. "Will I get to be a parent? What kind of parent will I be? Can I separate from my own parenting and be different? Can I become the perfect parent I want to be, and not the one I've been rebelling against all this time? If I'm no good as a parent, will I have impaired this baby?"
>
> Every mother and father dreams about [an] impaired baby. It is a rehearsal for what they might do if the baby is born impaired. They are preparing unconsciously for the impaired baby, and consciously for the perfect one. Somewhere

> in this ambivalence, anxiety and turmoil, a major purpose is served—to help the two extremes come together to work towards a mother-infant adjustment at the new birth. (Brazelton 1988)

As Brazelton's talk emphasized, there are characteristic mood swings from pleasure at the imminent possibility of her baby's reality to unconscious anxiety that either she or the baby may die at birth.

## WHAT IS A DYNAMIC?

When a baby is born, and in the first year of life, Mahler, Pine and Bergman (1975) recognized there was a repeat of the autistic, symbiotic, hatching, differentiating, and separating out. In therapy, the therapist helps these stages to continue in their normal course, like freeing mercury in a thermometer. Pregnancy is a series of ordered, primitive, potent psychic events, a foundation laid of a repeating dynamic. What is the predictive value in this? It is well documented that for each human the point of vulnerability or breakdown is different. Take a pregnant woman who is comfortable in the fusion stage but does not cope with the second-trimester differentiation. She will probably do fine when the baby is in the symbiotic phase after birth but may have difficulties as the baby develops autonomy.

### Preconceptive Ambivalence and the Dynamic of Wanting and Not Wanting a Pregnancy

Concepts of pregnancy, birth, and parenting, as well as sexuality, are alive and well throughout childhood. Each child, male and female, write their own individual internal drama of the creation of an infant. This is made up of their personal childhood experiences, their inner world life, and the phantasies their parents have consciously and unconsciously given them. A child fantasizes about having babies. Questions about babies—"Can I have one? With whom? How? When?"—will occupy phantasy and play through dolls and cars and other toys or symbols from a very early age (Kestenberg 1956). Before an infant is conceived there is a vast array of confusing and conflicting emotions in the infant's parents, resulting from internal world objects born from their attitudes to sexuality that developed during their childhood. Preconceptive ambivalence is the most significant source and model of ambivalence present in each of us in every stage of development and continuing through the whole of life. Birth is the climax but not the beginning of a continuum that starts at the preconceptive stage. Feder (1980) calls the ambivalence of mother and father towards conception "the evidence of procreative joy" as opposed to "procreative panic." The way the pregnancy progresses will affect these feelings. However, "the mutually attracted heterosexual couple awaken and stimulate in each other a series of interpersonal, ambivalent and contrary conflicts, usually unconscious" (Feder 1980, 162). They have their respective dilemmas towards pregnancy. There is both a fear and also a wish surrounding a pregnancy. The infant will be the highly vulnerable recipient of these ambivalences concerning sexual and erotic needs. These preconceptive ambivalences from the parents' childhood may be abortive, reparative, phallically or anally sadistic, joyful, or mournful due to object loss. They are different for each person. The internal representations of their parents, their own childhood experiences and environment affect these ambivalences. Feder states that "the parents' ambivalence as external objects determine the child's psychological and characterological destiny, eventually sensed, incorporated, repeated and perpetuated by the child now turned parent throughout generations. It stems originally from external reality; it is eventually incorporated and its origin unrecognised in the unconscious" (Feder 1980, 163).

In my study of twenty pregnant couples, I found those most able to tolerate their ambivalences during pregnancy were more positive and less anxious when their baby was born. No infant is wanted totally. The dynamic of wanting and not wanting one's offspring continues throughout the mother's, father's, and infant's life, seeking at each stage a psychic resolution. Here then is the paradox of the unborn child. Conceived in ambivalence, surviving or not surviving in the womb in ambivalence, and born into ambivalence. The life force is so strong and yet so vulnerable to opposite forces, an expression of the problem of conflict in human life.

## The Dynamic of the Dream, the Dread, and the Reality

There are three separate paths existing throughout life that are repeated at every phase. There is a dream of what the parents want their baby to be, the opposite which is the terror of what he or she might be, and in pregnancy, there is the unknown. Who is this baby? The parental mythology of the purpose of this baby's coming formulates itself in their minds during pregnancy. Is he going to be the fulfillment of their love? (He is the pronoun used for the infant in this chapter.) Is he going to be the declaration of their right to impulsiveness in their sexuality? Is he their sin, their punishment? Is he the embodiment of their evil or their virtue? The children of Holocaust victims were sometimes identified as perpetuating the Jewish race and preserving it from death. The migrant infant often had the role of fulfilling a parent's dream of greatness in a new country. Such mythological expectations affect the parents' perceptions of their child and their expectations. All infants carry some parental myth. The baby's birth can be a disappointment for a mother and a time of exultation. Here is the baby as he is, not the phantasy only, but now in reality. I have seen in my work that at every stage, past unconscious emotions are awakened, revived dreams, hopes and fears from the past return, and the parents will have another chance in their own lives to work through the same stage of development as their infant is working through. This is no less so during the growth phase of the embryonic and fetal infant.

## The Dynamic of Being and Reacting

Being and reacting are opposite to each other. In reacting, being is lost. Bion (1977) and Winnicott (1984a) speak of a state of being before birth, where no action or response is needed. Everything is provided. With the propulsion of birth, the infant is forced to react, and loses being, only to regain it again after birth. Here is another lifetime dynamic of being one's self, and losing one's self. In reacting and regaining one's self, Bion (1977) called the center of self "O" and gave the infant an ego "O" before birth. If there is trauma, the psychic pain is too severe. Even in utero, self can be lost.

## The Dynamic of Fullness and Emptiness, The Normal Narcissism of Pregnancy

A baby's kick, a baby's movement reassures a pregnant woman that she is full of life. For the pregnant woman there is a sense of superiority and elation of being full of penis?, breast?, baby? She feels she has everything. As Lemoine-Luccioni (1987) writes, paraphrasing Luke 1:42, she experiences herself as "full of grace, blessed among women and blessed in the fruit of her womb." After birth is a depression as if mourning the loss of that fullness. If the baby is healthy and feeding, reality wins. A new stage of symbiosis begins. This is the dynamic of the movement from healthy pregnant narcissism to the actual baby, and acceptance of it (Lemoine-Luccioni 1987).

## The Dynamic of Primary Maternal Preoccupation, Primary Maternal Protection and Primary Maternal Persecution

In the inner world of archaic objects ever present in our minds are dual opposites. Present and conscious in pregnancy is the phantasy of an evil mother who will rob the womb or kill the baby. The opposite is also present. There is the image of a mother who will protect from all harm, be omnipotent in shielding the infant, and powerful in protecting the mother-infant duo. The lack of control over what is growing inside the woman, be it a Christ child or a monster, heightens her fear of negative and persecutory forces as well as of benign positive ones. Both idealizing and negative forces may be projected onto her real mother, mother-in-law or husband. The fetus is not safe from projections either. He may be seen in turn as the savior of the family or as a foreign intruder ready to tear the mother's womb apart and endanger her life. These opposites of primary maternal persecution and primary maternal protection are dealt with by the mother in a stage towards the end of pregnancy and immediately after birth, known as primary maternal preoccupation.

## The Dynamics of Chaos and Order

As noted above, the three main stages in a woman's life where she experiences deep emotional and physical changes are the onset of puberty, pregnancy and menopause. Dinora Pines speaks of the third trimester of pregnancy:

> [This stage] is marked by bodily discomfort and fatigue. [There is a] need for mothering. . . . Memories of sibling rivalry seem to come to the fore and may be passed on to in-laws or old friends. There are characteristic mood swings from pleasure at the imminent possibility of her baby's reality, to unconscious anxiety that either she or the baby may die at birth. However strongly the outside world reassures her, the anxieties persist and there can be revivals of old guilts as to whether she can produce anything good or not. There is a beginning of impatience and drive to accomplish the task of birth and have her baby. There is a kind of feeling of exhilaration at being able to play an active role once more and surrender the passive one. (Pines 1972, 336–37)

The preoccupation of this final semester is so great and so intense that Winnicott (1984a) says if a baby were not there the mother would be considered mad. There are some mothers who, because of severe deprivation in their own childhood, cannot move into preoccupation. There are others who have entered it, and find great difficulty in moving out. They suffer from postnatal depression. In pregnancy, there is an inward turning that has the quality of a depressive state. This is quite different from postnatal depression because far from crippling, it is creative: far from blinding, it allows insight, and far from creating intolerable psychic pain, it will enable psychic pain to be processed and suffered. This adjustment between the dynamics of hope and despair, of dreams and reality, of joys and fears, continues throughout the parents' and baby's life together. Brazelton and Cramer's (1990) findings were that these parents interviewed in the months after their infant's birth had found a new order and structure and were considered normal. Out of the chaos the mother and father, initially fragmented, begin a newly defined identity. This is, of course, massively affected and intruded on by the infant's being, and by undertaking the responsibilities and demands of parenthood.

### The Dynamic of Knowing and Unknowing

A woman in pregnancy faces a very long period of unknowing. In the inexorable process of development over which she has no influence, she must tolerate changes that are beyond her control. As the baby is born, she begins to know and not know her baby. That dynamic of knowing and not knowing is one she lives with for the rest of her life. No mother truly knows her baby. She moves between knowing and not knowing as a dynamic from the beginning to the end.

## COUNTERTRANSFERENCE DURING PREGNANCY

The countertransference with which the therapist may have to deal in working with a pregnant woman is difficult and complex. Rivalry and envy may be aroused. The more unacknowledged by the therapist, the more it will intrude on the therapeutic process. There may be some forgotten or repressed element of one's own pregnancy, or desires to be pregnant that are invoked once more by the presence of a pregnant woman. Sympathy, empathy and protectiveness may well be present as the therapist becomes pregnant with the expanding patient. She may nourish her with emotional transfusions and interpretations, distilled perhaps from her own pregnancy and her own training. The therapist has two patients—the mother and her fetus—and feelings alternate for one or the other. There is a fine balance in elucidating the pathological while preserving those elements of idealization and phantasy that arc necessary for the future welfare of the baby and mother. Thus, every mother needs to remain under the impression that her baby is the best. It is through this capacity for idealization and a narcissistic identification with her baby that she will manage to achieve the never-ending sacrifices and continuous negotiation of painful conflicts and difficulties from infancy to adulthood and beyond. Finally, the fact of birth resulting from a pregnancy—the actual presence of a real and alive infant, no longer a dream, a phantasy, but a real baby—brings pride, pleasure and anticipation. This overwhelming adult achievement gives the push into coping with the realities of parenthood.

# Chapter 3

# Trauma During Pregnancy

How do past unresolved conflicts intrude on the present for a pregnant woman and her partner? Experiences and inner-world phantasies from infancy, childhood and adolescence are awakened during pregnancy and birth. Every emotion the pregnant woman has experienced as a baby, as a child, and as an adolescent as coming from her own mother—be it loving and adequate, or uncaring and neglectful, be it exciting or depressing, accepting or rejecting—goes into her vast unconscious storehouse of experiences. These become one of the main determinants of the kind of mother she experiences herself as. From her own feeding as a baby, toileting, loving, and hating her mother, feeling dependent on her, trying to establish independence, rivaling her for father's love, or seeking out her own sexual identity, come the resolutions that help her find her identity as a mother. Significant also are her relationships with her father, her siblings, and her friends.

The discussion in this chapter is informed by over one hundred interviews the author carried out with both pregnant women and their partners. (Anonymized excepts from these interviews are used to illustrate the main themes.) The importance of the partner cannot be overstated. However, because this is a book focusing on a woman's internal world during this time, it does mean the partner is not given the value he deserves. In our modern world the husband and wife can interchange roles, and each benefits from their sharing and interchanging roles.

## CHILDHOOD SEXUAL PHANTASIES

For the child, there is confusion about sexuality and babies, often "Who has what?" is not very clear either, and questions about "What is that for?" also abound. There is confusion between having a penis and having a baby, doing a pooh and having a baby, and between a vagina and a baby. Sexual excitement is undifferentiated. It can be oral, anal, or clitoral. Often sexual phantasies enacted with family members can be about domination and enslavement or ruling and being ruled. The "make-believe" arena gives boundaries to the sexual excitement, and play can be a protection against reality, while still expressing and sorting out phantasies of an unconscious nature. Fairy tales and drama enactments can carry a large amount of the excitation and resolutions of a little girl's own internal drama. The prince falls in love with the beautiful young princess, the prince finds the left-out unhappy Cinderella, the prince kisses the princess on whom a spell has been cast by a wicked witch and she wakes up to love and marry him. The variations are endless. Most often, a child's sexuality is translated into the area of play. Here the phantasies of having a baby to daddy, of rivaling and replacing mummy in his affection, of being already grown up, can be enacted in the safety of play with dolls and other toys. Each little girl writes her own internal drama out of the combination of the fabric of her own inner needs and the external messages from the mother, father and family around her. It is this, her internal drama, that will most affect her feelings about herself as a pregnant woman and an adult.

All the experiences, hopes and fears of early childhood become heightened in adolescence. It is a time of experimentation as to who she is, how she is as a sexual woman, and who and how she is as an adult. In the resolution, she can combine sexuality, aggression, and love. She can share with a partner and still insist on her identity as a woman. In her unconscious psychic structure, enormous changes are taking place. There is hopefully the fusing of all her childhood sexual areas—oral, anal, and clitoral—into her body. The same event is occurring psychically,and its emotional counterparts are finding their place too in her inner world. She overcomes the fear and hopefully finds the joy of intercourse and, in so doing, is able to own her own female sexuality. This is the model. There are so many variables. All too often, emotions and conflicts unresolved from the past and traumas in the present can unite to have a women experience her sexuality as fearful and disturbing to her. The lack of resolution of adolescence plays a particularly significant role in pregnancy and birth.

> Everything I spent my adolescence rebelling against seems to have come home to roost. I wanted to make sure I would never be like my mother; no one would ever trap me like she was trapped. I hated her for being so weak. Now I feel entrapped and just as weak. I just can't see the strong side of pregnancy or motherhood . . . I think because my father was such a bully and so dominating. He robbed my mother of any mind of her own. I am continuously frightened Tom will do the same to me. Now I'm pregnant, I keep thinking he already has. (Excerpt from research interview)

> I always sensed a deadness inside me, as if my mother was not alive to me. She was always depressed. Never happy. Will I "not be there" for my baby? I decided not to work and be home for him. Then I thought but my mother was always home. She just wasn't there. She was too depressed. Now I am starting to feel depressed and afraid I'm repeating history. (Excerpt from research interview)

In adulthood a woman's childhood desire to have a baby is freed of the incestuous possessiveness of wanting her father for herself. She looks toward a "real" partner of own. Her deep wish to have a baby is possible. Sexuality is acceptable. Her partner is acceptable. Her wish can be fulfilled. This gives her satisfaction and a sense of fulfillment in being pregnant, even as it awakens past unresolved conflicts with her mother, father, and siblings. The importance of the time of pregnancy for correcting past misconceptions cannot be overemphasized, as pregnancy and birth bring all these past feelings to the surface again. Many women during pregnancy hate themselves for feeling that they are becoming like their mothers who they have spent their life rebelling against. The fear of their mother can surface from their childhood unconscious as someone who wants to abort their babies and rob them of them, as someone who would rob them of their individuality, and as someone who desires to retain all the adult woman's power. There are deep unconscious phantasies of competitiveness and envy. Pregnancy, after all, signals the end of being a free person and the beginning an irrevocable lifelong tie as a mother to a baby. Some women express resentment toward their mothers for being a woman. Others are grateful for their identity in a way they had not experienced before.

> Jane had five abortions from aged 18 to 35. She had never wanted to have children as a result of an alcoholic father and because she was closely bonded to her mother, speaking to her every single day. Her grandmother's death gave her a feeling of wanting to have a child of her own in a very strong way. She had done everything possible to make sure the pregnancy was going to be all right. When she became pregnant, she came to see me, terrified that she would now be punished for her sins of the past "murders" as she called them and robbed of this baby that she now truly wanted. There was a far greater terror as she moved into therapy: this was a terror of an internal murderous mother who would punish her for wanting babies of her own and being separate from her. The abortions in the past had been a kind of effort to separate out from her mother and rival her, and then an effort to atone to the mother by aborting her babies. Now she was going to separate out she was terrified of the consequences. Her pregnancy which could have been such a time of fulfillment and joy became a time of terror. (Excerpt from case notes)

## TRAUMA OF HAVING A PREVIOUS INFANT WITH PHYSICAL, GENETIC, OR RETARDATION PROBLEMS

By becoming pregnant again a woman and her partner can awake the trauma of having a previous infant with physical, genetic, or retardation problems. A woman and her partner who already have a baby with a hereditary defect, suffer considerable apprehension and fear of repetition in a new pregnancy. It is all the more worrying because their fear of repetition has its basis in reality. The genetic determinants require thorough investigation and full discussion with the parents. The choice of becoming pregnant then becomes an educated one with a full understanding of the risks involved.

There are many different causes of hereditary problems. The two most common are hereditary disorders transmitted through autosomal recessive gene defects and the sex-linked dominant gene. In the first, the mother and father are both carriers. Neither have the illness themselves. With every single pregnancy, there is a one in four chance that the baby will have the defect. There is a two in four chance that the baby will be a carrier but will not have the illness. The fourth chance is that the baby will neither have the defect nor be a carrier. There is precisely the same risk with each pregnancy. In the second form, the sex-linked dominant gene, the female is the carrier and all the female offspring will be carriers, but will not have the defect. All the males will have the defect, but will not be carriers. They will not transmit the disease to their offspring, but the females will. Every couple needs a clear enunciation of the risks. Their decisions to try again can then be made on the basis of knowing the chances and risks involved. There are some cases where the answers are not so obvious, and this makes it even harder for the couple to make a choice. For couples who have chosen to risk another pregnancy, it can often be an emotionally difficult time. Being the transmitter of a hereditary defect can create unconscious feelings of guilt and a sense of being bad because one has "bad" genes. Our unconscious minds own responsibility for everything, even our genes, as if we had the omnipotent power to make them otherwise. Professional support may be needed as well as help from those around them during the pregnancy. They also need help if they choose not to have more children in order to mourn this loss.

> I feel guilty most of the time. Did I do this? Did I cause my baby's illness? Do I have a right, to take this risk with another one? Sometimes I try to say, "it's all his fault." If I had married someone else, this would never have happened. I know the facts, but I keep changing them in my mind. We decided to have another baby. Now I'm pregnant, we are wondering whether it was a selfish choice and whether we have a right to take such a risk of inflicting an illness on our baby. It's an awful strain on our marriage. We feel like criminals colluding

> in some crime. I worked so hard the whole pregnancy. I just made sure I kept busy and didn't think of the pregnancy at all. I had the most terrible dreams! Tom and I just weren't with each other. We were too frightened to let each other know how we felt. "I think every woman in the world is enjoying her pregnancy and I'm loaded up with terror half the time. It is not fair. Why me? What have I done? Can you imagine the fear of spending nine months to produce a source of grief and heartache for the baby and my husband and I. Dear God, be kind! Let this one be all right! (Excerpt from research interview)

> She was a normal baby! We were overjoyed. But I didn't know I would feel resentment towards her for being normal when the other one wasn't. I was lucky I had therapy and I could work through some of the feelings. Tom attached to the other one, feeling this one was all right so she didn't need him so much. It causes changes to your whole family pattern. (Excerpt from research interview)

A male partner's suffering is poorly acknowledged by the world around him. He, too, is afraid and has very little support in this, often being called on to be the strong one. It is just as great a threat to his self-esteem to have a child with an illness. He, too, mourns the loss of the healthy child.

## THREAT OF A MISCARRIAGE

Emotional strain is placed on a pregnant woman if she has a threat of miscarrying. Her central focus and preoccupation is the survival of the fetus. She may feel powerless to ward off danger and damage to her baby. There may be unconscious guilt that it would be her fault. She may involve herself in magical thinking, imagining she would cause it by something she does, something she eats, a cold she has, or even a walk she takes. She desperately looks for a cause that will make some sense of it for her. Is there an ill omen she should heed? She is helpless to do anything about the situation.

The normal fear of miscarriage that every pregnant woman may experience can develop out of all proportion. One mother said, "I became obsessed with the thought that this would be my punishment for rebelling as a teenager and for hating my own mother." Another became deeply aware of her ambivalence towards her unborn baby and felt this may be the cause of the threat of miscarriage.

> I was really upset when 1 found out I was pregnant again. I already had two children and was not planning any more. I've been in hospital since the fourth month. At first I even found myself wishing I could lose the baby. I wouldn't be sick any more if I lost it. Then I'd feel guilty for having thoughts like that. Then I'd think what if he survives, and then there's something wrong with him. I've been a lot worse since he's started to move, because I have started to feel motherly and protective. Once you can feel a little person in there, it's worse because you want him, so the fear of losing him gets worse. (Excerpt from research interview)

One woman I interviewed was physically ill for the whole of her pregnancy and constantly threatened with the possibility of a miscarriage.

> l felt inferior to other women. They could carry their babies OK. Why couldn't I? l am having terrible dreams of him being snatched through my stomach walls. I bet you think I'm a bit mad. I feel if l lost this baby, I'm a failure and everyone will know it. Sometimes, I talk to him and say, "don't let me down!"—as if he had control. (Excerpt from research interview)

A pregnant woman with a threatened miscarriage needs a great deal of support. She needs the extreme sensitivity and lability of her emotions understood, not only by her partner and family, but by the medical staff. Doctors need to explain the medical details of the situation, as thoroughly as they understand them, to her and her partner, several times if necessary.

## EXPERIENCE OF A PREVIOUS DEATH OF A BABY, AN ABORTION OR A MISCARRIAGE

When a pregnant woman has had a previous baby die, an abortion, or a miscarriage, this previous emotional trauma is reawakened in a most powerful way, by her present pregnancy. It is as if the trauma is not just remembered but relived. ln a psychic way it occurs again. So great is the phantasy of repetition, that at the point of crisis she does not differentiate one pregnancy from another.

> "This pregnancy seems just fine," the doctor told the mother. "Are you sure?" the mother asks. "The baby's alive? It"s alive?" She asks again. "Yes. It is," the doctor reassures her. She needed to be told, as if this one and the other had

> become mixed up in her mind. Even then she needed the constant reassurance of the baby moving to be sure. She later said, "Even when I was relieved, there was always in my mind the thought that I could be going through this again for nothing." (Excerpt from case notes)

A loss of a baby, a miscarriage, or an abortion leaves a scar for the rest of a woman's life. One older woman reported bursting into tears as she flew over a part of India where she had been a doctor and had lost her baby, twenty years before. She says she was not even thinking of it at the time. Pregnancy is not just a time when new deep wounds of a lasting nature can occur. It is a time when old wounds can have some healing. A dead baby cannot be replaced by having another one. Neither can a miscarriage. Each pregnancy is a unique experience. There is immense healing however when the previous psychic pain suffered can be relieved by a new healthy experience of a baby surviving and being well.

## TRAUMATIC LOSS OF A PARTNER DURING PREGNANCY AND EARLY AFTER BIRTH

Pregnancy is a vulnerable time. A pregnant woman's partner and family of origin, particularly her mother, take on new importance in protecting and caring for her as a mother with her beginning baby. Their emotional importance is as a direct result of her increased dependence. The loss of a partner through separation is hard enough to cope with, but loss through death becomes a real tragedy. Mourning during pregnancy cuts across her process of bonding with the unborn baby and can create chaos and confusion as she loses her protector, and the father of her baby. Self-blame for the loss is profound. Sometimes the loss is even blamed on her pregnant state or on the unborn baby in subtle ways that the woman herself hardly perceives. It may add to her terror of losing her baby since the issue of death as a possibility becomes so real to her. She might even bond with her baby as a defense against loss and mourning. In this way it meets her own needs more than the baby's needs. The baby's presence may be used to defend against psychic pain, or she may be so emotionally depressed she forgets the baby is there. For some pregnant women, there is the burden of carrying on with life for the baby's sake, when all she wants to do is mourn:

> I saw this woman when her son began day nursery. Her husband had been killed four years ago. She was very depressed, had been out with no one since and kept to a group of friends who looked after her. She had wanted to die herself when he died. Everyone had kept saying "think of the baby." Now with her son separating out and going to nursery, the shock of her husband's death was before her. She told me for months after his death, she had set the table each day for two, pretending that he was coming home. She still had his clothes in the drawers and hanging in the wardrobe. She told me too how she had not been to the funeral, had never visited his grave. She was completely bound to her in-laws as if making up for his absence by constantly giving them charge of her little boy. Once she began to mourn, she went to the funeral emotionally, in the sessions. She could cry for him for the first time. The pain had been too great before. She decided to visit his grave and lay flowers on it She was able to see her unconscious guilt in turning in on her pregnancy was unreal and had not caused his death. It became obvious that his death and her baby's birth had become mixed up in her mind. She would start to tell me about the death and ended up telling me about the baby's birth. It seemed during this therapy as if she was born herself and could go on to marry and have more children. (Excerpt from case notes)

This case illustrates the powerful effect of loss and the long-lasting effects it can have on a pregnant woman and her consequent relationship with her baby.

## THE CULTURE OF POVERTY

Some of the pregnant women I saw had to struggle heroically with problems to do with poor initial supports from their own mothers in childhood. They had serious marital problems, sometimes a previous miscarriage, or a previous baby die, or a baby born with hereditary illness, or some abnormality. Deserted by their partners, with other small children, and financially destitute, their pregnancies could never for them be anything more than barely being able to survive. Many lacked the support of a mother or other family or friends.

This next case study is about J., a mother who lives in an inner-city suburb. I initially met J. through my research but she later became a patient due to her circumstances.

> I am thirty-four years of age. I have been separated from my husband for six months now. I have three daughters, ages nine, eight and seven, and a son aged ten weeks. My husband left me when I was pregnant with this last baby. It was an unplanned pregnancy. There were lots of rows and loss of temper on both parts. I pleaded for him to stay, he insisted I had let him down and had tricked him into this pregnancy. I had an IUD and the pregnancy was an accident. He doesn't believe me. The doctor removed the IUD after I got pregnant. It left me

with what the doctor called an irritable uterus. I was hospitalized three times during my pregnancy and my children had to fare for themselves with my husband looking after them. The last time I came home from hospital, he left. I felt it was the [unborn] baby's fault.

I didn't want this baby and I've had nothing but trouble with him from the day he was born. I was depressed right through my pregnancy. I am still irritable and unhappy most of the time. I can't get away from this baby waking up and crying. From the beginning he has refused to suck and every feed is a nightmare. I have a two-bedroom house. I have three girls and my son is in their room. They all complain they have no space of their own. When he is sleeping the girls can't make any noise or even move around, because if he wakes up, no one sleeps. I moved him in with them because I hadn't slept for nights and l was afraid, I would hurt him.

I have money problems, big ones. I sometimes don't have enough money for food. My parents won't help because my husband fought with them and I took his side before he left. The girls loved their father and their grandparents and they've lost both. The girls school work is going down. The teachers are complaining. They won't let me tell the teachers their father has left. I imagine they still want to protect him.

I just keep hoping he'll come back. I have to, it's all I've got to look forward to. l feel it can't get any worse. I'm depressed most of the time. I suffer from terrible headaches. I need someone to look after me, not me look after children. I think I've just got to make it through today and tomorrow might be better. (Excerpt from research interview and case notes)

J. is in need of help—now. She needed help more when she was pregnant, as did her partner. She desperately needed to feel wanted during her pregnancy. Her husband's rejection of her is equated with his rejecting the baby inside her. It is very hard to love an unborn baby, part of herself, when she feels rejected and unwanted because of it. It seems the baby's feeding and sleeping problems were both his, and his mother's, cry of distress and a cry for help. Her attachment to him has been severely disturbed, first by the pregnancy not being wanted and then by the trauma of her husband's leaving. A pregnant woman is as vulnerable as a fetal infant, she needs nurturing herself if not from a partner than from family and friends. J. had none of these supports. The one thing that held her through when I spoke to her after was the support of her social worker. She said, people asked her if she felt so negatively, why didn't she abort. She looked so depressed as she said, "and do to him what my husband did to me."

L. is a young suburban mother. Her burden seems more than anyone can or should have to carry.

I am twenty-eight years of age. I have a daughter aged three and a son aged two. When my husband and I found out our second baby had cerebral palsy it was

> too much for him to cope with. He left home supposedly to work in the country. He never was one for responsibility in the first place. He came back when the baby was eight months old. Everything looked good for a couple of months. When I found out I was pregnant again, he left again. I've been on my own for the whole pregnancy. It's been a nightmare. I'm terrified something will be wrong with this pregnancy like with my last baby. I have nightmares every night thinking this one is going to be like the last one. The last one was premature and I keep looking for signs of this one being premature. I became such a nervous wreck with constant headaches I just couldn't cope anymore and I moved in here with my mother and my brother. She doesn't want me here. She tells me so at least twice every day. I can't stay here. My husband will never come back if I stay here. I've got a dollar to my name and my welfare check isn't due until next week. I can't even afford a newspaper to look for a flat, let alone a house. My husband contacted me last week. He said he'd come back when this baby is born. Look we don't love one another, but I've got to be practical. I need him. I can't even get to the doctor every fortnight for the other little one with cerebral palsy. I'm going to make sure I don't attach to this baby when its born. I'm frightened I will attach to him and break my heart again, like I did when I found out Tom had cerebral palsy. I'm going to make sure he's all right first, before I let myself feel anything. (Excerpt from research interview)

## THE SINGLE WOMAN

More single women are choosing to be pregnant. Some choose motherhood before it is too late. They may prefer a father's presence, but decide to have a baby without the support of a partner, rather than miss the experience. As one woman told me, "I was getting older. I didn't have a permanent partner, but I desperately wanted a child of my own. I knew it was now or never." Some (single) lesbians also wish desperately to have an infant. Being lesbian does not exclude the desire to be a mother.

All single women interviewed highlighted the difficulties of being pregnant and single. They saw themselves as disadvantaged. In the absence of support and protection there was a need to be tough and they saw illness and vulnerability during pregnancy as a luxury. They felt society had moved away from the moral code of the undeserving single mother, but had done nothing to support her. If a single woman chooses to keep her baby, she should manage on her own and not burden the community seems to be the most common dictum.

For C. the transition to adolescence and the transition to motherhood coincided. She had been adopted as an infant. She saw pregnancy as a way of filling the emptiness of abandonment and the lack of real affection in her home life. It may have been a way of finding her real mother. In keeping her baby she may have been fulfilling her fantasy of what she wished her mother had done with her.

> The most important thing in my life is that I was adopted. I was told about it much too early, and I spent my childhood crying about it. My brother was adopted too, but it didn't seem to affect him in the same way. I moved down to Sydney to work as a nanny when I was seventeen. I got pregnant to Greg. Greg, said, "I'm not ready to be a father," and just went walkabout, like mum and dad predicted he would. I wanted this baby which I was sure was a boy so much, but I got really depressed while I was pregnant. I thought, what have I done? It scared me heaps. My body was changing, before my eyes. I didn't look so good any more. There was a baby in there and I was going to have it. What a responsibility! I felt I could hardly look after myself, let alone a baby. I had made the decision to go on with it myself and there was no way I was going back on it. I went with guys I wouldn't normally have gone out with. I needed more desperately than ever for someone to love me. I kept dreaming Greg would come back and we would make a go of it. He was in my mind the whole pregnancy as the father of my baby, but as a dream, a fantasy. It's not reality. I knew it wouldn't work even if he did come back. I was adopted as a baby. My real mum was only sixteen, same as me. I fantasied a lot about her while I was pregnant. I thought, she had to give me up, there was nothing else she could do. There was no care for unmarried mothers in those days. I was needing a mother to cuddle and hold me. My adoptive parents were so cold and judging of me, I said to myself, "My real mother would have cuddled me!" I think I had that baby so I could make up for what I had missed. Something of mine that I could just love for myself. It's a selfish thought, because, oh boy, you sure don't know what you are in for. When I had her it came to me so simply. I'm responsible for this little baby. That responsibility won't end until the day I die. She's not here for me she's here for her. (Excerpt from research interview)

## MIGRATION

A migrant pregnant woman has particular problems. The migrant man and woman suffer the trauma of identity loss in the migratory process. They no longer know where they belong or who they are. They often lose social status, and social and personal orientation. A migrant family is not on holiday or even just transferring from one country to another. For the refugee, there is a wrenching from a familiar culture known since birth to a culture that is alien and where they will never feel they fully belong. They often lose their family also, and are wrenched from a village environment of emotional caring to an environment that sees them as inferior at best and has no concern or acknowledgment of them at all at worst.

Pregnancy is a migratory process of an internal kind. Combined with the trauma and chaos of external change in migration, the stresses are enormous. Add to this the different cultural patterns, sometimes isolation, loss of the husband to more work and more time away from home, and the strain can become too much to bear.

A. is a young Lebanese woman, who found the transition from her country of origin to her new country to be an immense strain and a loss of status. Her story is not different to that of many others. She is a typical migrant from a little village in the mountains, and the transition to the city is also hard for her to encompass.

> In my village if you are pregnant, you are a very important person. Motherhood is a big thing. It is what every woman longs for. No one cares here. Even my husband doesn't care so much. I think he is worried because it means I don't go to work as much with a baby and we need the money. I am missing my mother and my aunts and my cousins so much. They would have had such good help to give me and already they are very happy when we tell them, but they are sad because they cannot help. There are a lot of our Lebanese friends here, but they all go to work like I did. I would rather sit under our olive tree and just live on dry bread and olives and know I could stay with my baby than be here and know I have to give him to someone else to mind and go back to work. I've been looking at working at home and there is a lot of this work, but you can go all day and they pay you almost nothing. They know they have you caught because you want to stay with your baby and you need the money so what can you do. I'm frightened about the birth because I hate the hospital, and I will feel even more a stranger there. That is what it is like when I go there for a check-up. No one looks very happy; we line up and just wait. Mothers don't count in this country. I really want to go back home, but we will never be able to do that and my baby, when he is born, will think this is his country. It isn't mine and it never will be, in that way I will be a stranger to my own child. Back home we were poor but happy, here we are better off and our children will be better off, so what can we do. (Excerpt from research interview)

## REFUGEES FROM WAR AND TRAUMA

There are quite different problems for the person who leaves their country of origin because of political violence or war, than for those who migrate because of economic hardship. Not only have they been victims of war in their own country, but they are often exploited here. Pregnant women may work on machines in crowded rooms from morning until night for a salary that would shock any union member. Many people may live in a tiny house.

Their expectations of what to expect differ because of the hardship they have experienced. They are grateful to be in a safe country.

N. and his wife V. are such a couple. V. is in her seventh month of pregnancy. When I interviewed them, they had been in Australia for two months. The interview was in an outpatient section of a large city maternity hospital, because they were afraid to allow me to home visit. It was as if they were not yet sure they were safe here in Australia, nor even sure why we would want to hear their story. They feared they could be sent back and appeared bewildered and depressed, despite their constant expressions of relief. They told my interpreter that they feared not for themselves but for their family members who were still in in danger. N. and V. were happy to speak with me, once I explained that I would like to understand them better and give this understanding to others. There was a lack of enthusiasm and emotional affect in everything they told me. They were aware of, and responsive to my warmth and the welcoming friendly manner of my interpreter, but they were too emotionally damaged to be able to relate anything but events. It was the understatement of what they had been through that made this a different interview. There was a resigned matter of fact relating of events, for example, "We were put off our land with no belongings and no place to go. V. was three months pregnant. She miscarried on the way." They had been through too much, and were still dazed and bewildered. They presented an autistic response, born out of suffering more than was bearable. Although it seemed a haven of freedom here, the past was ever present. N. repeated ten times, they must now forget the past and live the lives they now had. "We must look only to the future," he said each time I asked him about his past.

> V: We did not come directly to Australia. We came from Hong Kong. We have been refugees there for three years. The first year was the worst, because we lived in a cage and could not go out anywhere. We were prisoners. I had already had three miscarriages. I knew I was too weak and sick to have another baby. This camp was not a good place to have a baby. I had an IUD put in when we arrived there.
>
> N: We had good land and we came from a hardworking and happy family. We grew rice. Both our families came from the same village. Both our families were very happy for us to marry because they had been friends for a long time. We were lucky not to be caught in any of the fighting during the war. We had our first son after only one year of marriage. Everyone celebrated with us. We did not go to a hospital but to our clinic. We had a midwife and he was very healthy. When he was two the soldiers arrived one day and said, "We want all this land for government use and you must leave it in two days." V. was pregnant three months. We had to leave all our belongings, because we could not carry anything. We walked to a city one hundred miles away. V. lost the baby on the way.

> It was very hard there and there was no work. V. lost another baby and she was very miserable and lost hope of a healthy baby.
>
> V: I felt very weak and very sick and each time I lost a baby I became sicker and more unhappy. We decided to flee with our parents to Hong Kong. My husband's brother had come to Australia two years before. We asked if he could bring us here. When we knew that we could come to Australia I took out the IUD and I became pregnant again. This was my new country baby and I knew here I would have a freedom baby here and it would be alright. I was five months pregnant when I felt the baby move. It was the week I arrived in Sydney. We do not choose a boy or a girl, just that it will be well and able to live here safely. I do not become sad when I think about the past, because I must forget it and not remember. Our baby will not know there was a past, but will only know this country. I miss my mother because she is not here now when I am pregnant. We do not write to our family back home, it is too dangerous. I write to my mother in Hong Kong. She is seventy years old. I do not cry because she is not here. We do not cry, N. and I. Our son also does not cry. We are happy here. (Excerpt from research interview)

N. and V.'s protestations of happiness seemed not to fit the grim expressions on their faces. I knew they did not cry because they were traumatized and no longer knew how to cry. I knew she would make a good and secure mother, and he would make a caring father. But I wondered how hard it would be to have a baby that shared none of their history, that had known none of their previous suffering or pain. I asked my interpreter, who was so lively by comparison, "Are all the refugees like this?" She said, "Yes, they are because they cannot believe this is real. They have had things too hard. Later, they will be alright and they will be able to laugh, and then they will be able to cry."

## THE RELEVANCE OF SUPPORT DURING PREGNANCY

The traumas presented in this chapter involve a psychic pain beyond what can be managed by the woman alone, or even with the support of a partner, family, and friends. Pregnancy is a time when old conflicts are awakened and when unconscious feelings are near the surface. For both partners emotional strains are increased by changes in their external and emotional inner worlds as they transition to parenthood.

The pregnant woman and her partner are highly motivated during this time to "get things right" in preparation for their baby's coming. This motivation is more significant than at any time in their lives. Professional help early can sometimes save later pain, conflict, and heartache. It can help the couple develop a healthy relationship for the future. Pregnancy is not only about producing a healthy baby but also a healthy mother and father. This becomes all the more important when it is understood that pregnancy is not only a preparation for motherhood or fatherhood but its basis. If the transition to motherhood and fatherhood becomes distorted, marital breakdown, postnatal depression, and many more problems may result. Some pregnant women cannot allow themselves to move into a regressed state and cope with the normal chaos and confusion this brings. They miss the normal emotional processes of pregnancy and are vulnerable to breakdown after birth. Some women become so immersed in the processes, they cannot make their way out of the normal depression and need help to enjoy their baby.

## *Chapter 4*

# Identifying and Working With Trauma During Pregnancy

Pregnancy is a sensitive period. Trauma occurs more potently than at other life stages. During normal maturational processes, there is a degree of chaos as the old order changes, giving place to new, pre-conceptive ambivalence, pregnancy, oedipal phase, latency, adolescence, marriage and motherhood, fatherhood, menopause and old age. Perhaps the most sensitive of changes is the time when the woman begins the maturational process into motherhood in pregnancy. Trauma during pregnancy seriously affects a woman's relationship with her infant, her partner, and her whole life with serious consequences. Experiences during pregnancy such as miscarriage, stillbirth, possible retardation, or social problems such as domestic violence create trauma that may have awful consequences if unresolved. This trauma may result in excruciating psychic pain, beyond what is bearable, and the woman's internal world may disintegrate, resulting in a total internal implosion. A barrier is created to protect against reaching that pain, and any links to the possibility of that pain are defended against with a resultant autistic deadened core which takes away the possibility of feeling. However, trauma can be relived in similar consequent events, exposing the pain and so creating a chance to work the trauma through more successfully. Reliving, if it fails to resolve the trauma, may make it worse.

To understand this further, there is a need to understand how an experience becomes a thought, and how it is stored for future use in the psyche and in the mind, how it moves from an experience with the emotional content saturating it, to a thought, an abstraction and then a model for future use. These processes of how an experience becomes a thought and eventually stores in the mind a model for future use come from Bion (1977). There are marked changes in the psyche's normal functioning created by trauma. Trauma affects the capacity to change an experience into an abstraction and then a model for further use. In trauma there is no movement to normal mind processes;

the experience remains the thing in itself. That means the experience cannot be stored in mind as a model for use in future living experiences; the whole experience is repressed. The psychic pain in trauma remains as a terror, a series of facts not saturated with meaning. The experience remains the experience in itself and is repressed as that. It cannot be thought, or even thought about, and so cannot move through the processes of realization, representation, model creation and abstraction, which means there is no model to store and to call on. It is as the experience in itself with all the emotions of the previous event, exactly as if they were remains frozen in time and space. In fact, there is no "before"; there is only "now." The ego to protect itself from unbearable pain and terror creates barriers to any link in this experience.

The deadening described by Edna O'Shaughnessy (1981) can sometimes go on for months, even years. The hidden reason behind the deadness is too terrible and painful to know psychically. It is the task of the therapist to tolerate this deadness, not judge it as hostility, or as good or evil, but to respect and recognize the intense pain and "frozen with fear" state behind it. The task of the health professional is physic understanding of this deadened space—experiencing it, receiving it from the patient, allowing minute amounts of the terror to emerge with sensitive timing, and returning it to the patient in a way that is digestible. This allows the experience to be thought while retaining the emotion attached to it, and so can be converted for future use as part of the psyche, so that life can return in minute experiences and eventually allow deadness to be replaced by an alive experience.

Frances Tustin extended this way of thinking about and treating traumatized patients. On reading my paper, "The Psychic Space in Trauma" (1991), she wrote to me personally each month and later developed a paper in which she included my thinking. In personal correspondence, she wrote:

> In Bion's theory of "reality" his emphasis was always "why now?" and continually on the "thing in itself." He saw reality as internal and external, as that which emerges from one's intuition and from the world around one. This is prominently featured in Bion's horizontal and vertical sections of the grid, as the sensory impulse is transformed from a beta element to an alpha element via a successful series of processes he documents in each square. The result of these processes is Bion's symbol "O" for truth. Truth allows mental digestion. Moving immediately from the sensory need to the action without thought is acting out and anti-truth. That separation between digestion and action is also the separateness between phantasy and reality, between dreams and wakefulness. It is the lack of this separation that occurs less in the neurotic, more in the borderline, and even more in the psychotic. (Frances Tustin, personal communication to author, 1992)

In our unconscious is a plethora of thoughts without a thinker waiting to be thought. However, which thoughts are thought, depends on external circumstances and internal needs. Inner and outer truth come together. This is "O," but truth is the "thing in itself." This has broken down entirely for the psychotic and less so for the neurotic. There are actual physical events, now well documented and researched, that show how in trauma that part of the mind which changes the experience of something into a thought or a realization is closed down and no longer works. The closing down between the hippocampus and the amygdala allows for action rather than thought, and the primitive fight or flight can occur to protect the person. In the next section, I present a case example, giving a real-life experience of trauma and recovery from it.

## DR. Q.

Some months after Dr. Q.'s baby had died within hours of birth, Dr. Q. presented for therapy. Her presenting symptom was depression caused by the loss and a feeling she would be unable to conceive again. She spoke in an odd, autistic-like, faraway manner. The colloquial term would be "spaced out." Dr. Q. was an older first-time mother, in love with her partner, and she had very much wanted this infant she had lost. The therapy was extremely difficult, and its effect amazed me. At times the strength of the repression was such that I felt out of touch, not only with her but also with myself. It was as if an iron shutter had been reached, and there was nowhere for me to go. At such times I thought crazy thoughts which had nothing to do with Dr. Q. or with any thinking of my own. These were fragmented, and I could not hold them. Sometimes I could not move or talk even though I wanted to. The effort seemed impossible. I always made time after her sessions to recover. It was helpful for me and for her, to experience these feelings. This dead space at first was the place we could not know, must not know, and later did know, and even later did know of the morass of primitive powerful feelings that exuded from it. These were not only of raging pain but phantasies of cold-blooded murder of her newborn by a destructive cruel mother inside her. She, as a mother, had died; her internal mother had died. She was both the murderer and the victim. Terrible things, unknowable things had happened as she moved from this dead space through a severe depression of self-blame, accusations of the doctors, the hospital, her partner, her real mother (who she had not seen or spoken to since that day), and finally me. It was I who was destructive and murderous and destroyed any life inside her.

During this period of our work, she became pregnant again. There were most powerful phantasies that I would take and kill this baby as her punishment for having it. This became hallucinatory with her sobbing about having to give the baby to me to avoid my killing it. She had phantasies of hiding it, dreams of smuggling it out under a pile of garbage on a truck from a dangerous village where I dwelt. These were so strong at times she feared to come to the session, terrified of the damage I might do. She sometimes clung to her husband, and at other times she wanted nothing to do with him. Likewise, with me, it changed often. Sometimes I was a positively hallucinated mother who would save her baby this time, but increasingly I became a persecutor who would destroy it.

In the sixth month of pregnancy, Dr. Q. took a long weekend break. During the first two days, she suspected the baby was not moving; by the end of the third day she was convinced it was dead in her womb. She was inconsolable, screaming and crying out that her baby was dead. Since she was herself a doctor and a specialist, her partner, confused at first, in the end believed her. He was distraught, more by her inconsolable state of anguish than the loss of the baby. She presented for her session ashen white. She told me her baby was dead inside her. She had screamed with anguish and unbelievable pain when she discovered it two days before, but now she was in quiet despair. She described how she had been in her bedroom and looked in the mirror and realized in seeing herself that her baby was dead. To my amazement, the conversation became confused, and I found she was telling not of this one but of the one that had died. She cried quietly as she told me every little detail of her first baby's death for the first time. Every moment of that fateful day was related, the medical procedures, the people who came to tell her of the death, and the unbearable pain she had felt, which she, as a doctor, must not show. As she was speaking, her voice became calmer, until she just lay there in silence for quite some time. Then she said quietly, "The baby just moved. I can feel movement!" She did not speak for the rest of the session as if absorbing the truth of the moment. She was able to mourn the death of the previous baby in the following months with me and was doing fine until the third trimester when her anxiety became overwhelming again. She needed, she said, to have the birth on her own, and exclude me from it. She returned after the birth. "I came to show you the baby," she said, seemingly well bonded with him. She paid money owed from before and left, not returning. Her baby lived, as did a subsequent infant.

When a woman's baby dies, this emotional trauma is awakened by a new pregnancy in a most powerful way (Lewis 1983). The experience is not just remembered, relived, or repeated, but seen as a continuation in time and space without differentiation. The dramatic moment of change was when Dr. Q. could separate out the dead baby from the alive one. It was with the narration, sharing the experience of the trauma with me and my receiving it, that allowed the change. The pattern is always the same: the dramatic breakthrough with unbearable suffering, the telling so simple, the submission to loss and then an acceptance of new life.

## THE AUTISTIC SPACE IN TRAUMA

This autistic core at the center seems similar to the empty space in autism. There is a hardness in the denial, yet also vague wafting, an "out of touch" feeling of non-presence paradoxically present in the sessions. The space is a "non-event" described by Lewis (1983) as a "no go" area. The reasoning behind the deadness is too terrible, too painful to know psychically. The massive primitive feelings made available when the deadening was disturbed also bear discussion. It was apparent in Dr. Q.'s therapy that confrontation with her loss of affect and with the loss of her alive internal objects was terrifying. With the loss of affect, emotional contact was lost for her when she most needed it. Frances Tustin (1990a, 105) says, "The bereft person is frozen with shock, is numb and dumb. . . . I have come to see that this state has been preceded by flaming and blinding rage about this disappointment. This has been unbearable because it has not been sufficiently received and understood. Thus, it seems to implode back on the child." So it is with unresolved trauma. Dr. Q. expressed her rage at her impotence and her sense of being helpless prey in the presence of a fate over which she had no control.

The person in unresolved trauma cannot occupy their own center stage to balance these primitive aspects of their personality. Hence there is left an unoccupied center, an empty stage, an autistic space. It was not until Dr. Q. could relate the trauma, the narrator of her own drama, and have it presented and heard, that the curtain on that drama could be drawn. Then the curtain could rise on the drama of the new life that had begun within her. Lewis and Casement (1986) stress that the event of pregnancy inhibits the process of mourning. Dr. Q could not get on with this pregnancy until she had separated it from the previous one. In pregnancy, internal objects and the internal physical baby become fused and confused. The pain in the trauma was too great to be borne . In each case, the alive presence of a "containing person or therapist" had to enter the dead space and experience it, and so show how to break out of it. The sessions in which the therapist was as if in an unbearable induced paralyzed state of being unable to move or be, mirrored her internal world. The breaking out of this space, enabled her to do so, and mourning could take place. There was a confusion between losing and finding, between life and death, and with that, there was no discrimination between time and space and persons. This pregnancy and the last one, this alive pregnancy and the previous dead infant, the boundaries between being alive and being dead herself were lost.

In healing there was a return of affect. The deadening or autistic space was identifiable: it was the acknowledging of it, the daring to experience it by the therapist that allowed her experiencing of the psychic pain and the resolution. Denial could be released and then repression freed, allowing remembering and knowing of what must not be known. However, it is impossible to assess how effective the healing was and how much residual damage was caused to her life with this infant and her relationship with it.

## IMPLICATIONS FOR THERAPEUTIC TECHNIQUES

The factors basic to the treatment of trauma are the experiencing of the autistic deadened space, by therapist and patient, the holding in it—interpreting it. For the therapist, there is the problem of combating forces to do with "what must not be known." With severely traumatized people, the understanding of what has happened to them may be more than the therapist can bear. Pontalis (1981, 196) writes, "Unconscious areas not even accessible consciously to the therapist are being worked on by the patient. These wounds open old sores, with unforeseen infiltrations which transverse and animate our psyche." Those people traumatized by such intrusion "touch us to the death" in an effort to secure our own psychic death, even as they are aware of the area of their own psychic death—attacks on linking become attacks on the therapist's effort to secure links.

The patient's incapacity to store, retain, and symbolize can often mean therapeutic efforts need to be repeated over and over. The therapist is viewed as a persecutor until the traumatized patient begins to accept the therapist as a holding, securing presence. Collusion between patient and therapist may occur against experiencing pain, against ambivalent and negative feelings in the transference and countertransference. Mutual idealizing denies the patient "*la douleur d'exister*." The patient is condemned to continued flight and defense, the alternative being a pain they fear cannot be held. The therapist needs to make that holding possible. Where there has been trauma, an acknowledgment of the real event is necessary; the reality factors need acceptance. Otherwise, the validity of affect is not acknowledged, and any interpretation is experienced as persecutory causing a serious empathic breakdown.

In Betty Joseph's paper "Towards the Experiencing of Psychic Pain" (1981, 100), there is a finely developed awareness of the patient who cannot be in pain and, therefore, cannot suffer it. She describes minute movements backwards and forwards towards the experience of psychic pain as a movement towards a psychic birth. She adds that pushing by unmitigated interpreting of good and evil may make things worse. Bion (1977, 19) says the traumatized person experiences "pain but not the suffering." He is in the pain, overwhelmed by it, the pain is not in him. How does this pain become an ego function, rather than the ego being overwhelmed? The answer is by allowing the pain of mourning to be lived with and suffered, not denied. The psychotherapeutic experience is a continuous movement from resistance to acceptance of daring to be in pain, and thence to experiencing and suffering one's own pain. In suffering pain, a thought process is required to integrate it.

The acknowledgement of having destroyed internal objects, in rage and anger at loss, allows love and hate to meet, with the ensuing true guilt of the depressive position (Winnicott 1965). Sometimes work on the autistic-like space may well require a more active role on the part of the therapist. The very act of waiting denotes a presence, hope, and willingness to take projections good and bad, of which the original space is devoid. The active acknowledgement of this space allows the patient's coming to life, as pain unbearable becomes pain suffered and hence tolerated.

## ACKNOWLEDGMENT

Norma Tracey (1991) "The Psychic Space in Trauma," Journal of Child Psychotherapy, 17 (2): 29–43., copyright © Association of Child Psychotherapists, reprinted by permission of Taylor & Francis Ltd, http://www.tandfonline.com on behalf of Association of Child Psychotherapists.

# *Chapter 5*

# The Psychic Pain of Trauma

## *Therapy Relating to Trauma During the Newborn Period*

The specific autistic-like space discussed in this chapter is caused by an excess of psychic pain flooding the ego, the failure of projective identification to find a holding container, and the loss, through rage, of good internal objects. This breakdown results in unthinkable fear, hence a loss of the capacity to think and to symbolize, and to suffer and process pain. Archaic denial takes the place of repression and there is regression to unconscious functioning, with the loss of secondary processing.

This is a theme repeated throughout this book. The many case studies describe this space and the breakdown in internal processes leading to it. Through these cases there is an attempt to define specific techniques by which the therapist or mother, through becoming a good-enough container, through having the capacity to wait in the space, through being able to tolerate the patient's projective identification, allows the unbearable pain to become bearable so that life can return. This case particularly deals with the unconscious processes so powerful in trauma that they deny life and confuse it with death.

### MR. AND MRS. WHITE

Mrs. White is thirty years of age. She has had premature twins, who she visited in the ward in the early days of their lives. Then at about eight days, one of the twins died. It was two weeks since the ward sister had seen Mrs. White in the ward. At first, in the ward team discussion, the thought was she might be mourning the first twin's death. However, she had not telephoned or come in by the second week, and the ward sister alerted the ward team, and we discussed how to approach this problem. The baby's medical prognosis was good. The team decided to invite the mother and father in for an interview, with me first and then include the occupational therapist and pediatrician. The parents canceled two appointments and came for the third. They had a child aged six at home and owned an early morning milk delivery service. They told me on the phone that they could not "make time" to come in, as they were very busy with the deliveries.

When they finally came to the interview, they were silent for some time as if wondering why they had been invited. When they began to speak, it was in a stilted and closed-off way. The father began to speak first, saying neither he nor his wife saw any purpose in seeing me. They had coped with the baby's death very well. As the interview progressed, I was more than a little surprised to note that they did not make any mention of the baby (the surviving twin) on the ward. The father explained how successful he had been in distracting his wife from her grief by involving her in the milk run, which used up all their time. He also had his hands full coping with his work. This had successfully taken their minds off the baby's death. She eventually said, "Yes, but we stay up till 2 a.m., and we begin the milk run at 4 a.m." I asked her if she was telling me that the distraction was not working. There was silence. They both looked stunned and sat silent and angry. "Four!" she called out loudly. "Four miscarriages! And now this!" She threw the words at me. I said, "This? Like yet another miscarriage?" "No! Worse! It is like I haven't had a baby. I haven't had anything." I said, "Are you telling me the pain of facing what you have had and lost is so great, you would prefer to deny you have had a baby at all?" Her husband looked forbiddingly at me as if to question what I was doing. Then she began to cry. They were angry tears. Slowly he began to cry. After a considerable time, I said, "Mr. and Mrs. White, there is still another baby alive on the ward." Eventually, the mother said, "We don't want to know!" I said, "I guess you are telling me the pain of loss is so great, you dare not take the risk of believing there is another alive baby for fear you may lose it also?" She nodded. "Perhaps it's easier not to know about life or death," I said, and we sat silently.

With their agreement, I then called the occupational therapist and the pediatrician. The occupational therapist arrived. "I have just come from your baby now," she said empathically. The mother responded by talking about her mother. "My mother is very ill in [the] hospital. I have had to keep up trying to visit her and cope with my father. She is too sick to know what is happening to us." I said that perhaps she was telling me the mother in her was too sick with grief to cope with the thought of the other baby. "Yes! I am coping with John (her husband) and my daughter Nell and our work. We look all right, but we feel dead, just empty inside." They seemed to sit with the emptiness.

The pediatrician arrived. The Whites began questioning the doctor, slowly at first and then it gained momentum. They were hostile questions at first but became eager and almost desperate. "What happened to Tom? Why didn't he live? What did you do wrong on the ward? Was it the hospital's fault? Was it our fault? We had handled him. We thought we had given him an infection or a virus. Sister had suggested we touch him. We wish now we hadn't." The doctor explained carefully and simply why the baby had died, and began to explain the difference between the dead baby and the alive one. He answered each of the mother's questions carefully. Her face became a little animated. "Is she moving?" she asked. "Quite a bit. She kicks quite strongly!" he said. "The sister told us on the phone she still had tubes down to feed her." "Yes, she has. We don't want to tire her out sucking." "Can she suck then?" "Oh yes. If you put your finger in her mouth, you'll see she sucks like a little race-horse." There was silence. "Does she move normally?" "Yes, she does. There does not appear to be any impairment." Finally, "Is she alive then?" "Yes, she is. Look, your baby is doing well. I cannot say for sure with a baby this small, but the chances are good. There is no sign of any damage at this stage. Would you like to see her?" She looked questioningly at her husband. "Well, I suppose we could just take a look. There is not much you can do while she is in an incubator, just look."

The occupational therapist took them over to the ward. She reported that when they arrived on the ward, they were diffident about going in. They stood by the crib, nervously watching their baby and commenting to each other on her appearance, her movement, and her breathing. They anxiously asked if it was uneven. The ward sister explained that it was no more than would be expected. The occupational therapist asked, "Would you like to touch her?" They carefully washed their hands. First mother, then father put hands in the crib and stroked the baby's hand. She grasped the father's finger tightly. Then the mother put her hand in again, and she held on to her finger. They were both very emotionally moved by the experience. The occupational therapist asked if they would like to hold the baby. The mother sat beside the crib, and the baby was placed in her arms. The mother's face lit up, as did the father's as he gingerly took his turn.

The mother came every day, all day, after that. This baby survived and went home with the parents.

## Discussion

Mrs. White saw all of her ills, her mother's illness, her four miscarriages, and the infant's death as caused by her. She feared they had killed one of the twins by touching him, and so feared they would kill the live one by touching her, or even acknowledging her as alive. In a desperate effort to find an answer where there was no answer, she pathetically seems to be quizzing the doctor, "Did you kill her, or did we?" If a therapist becomes caught up in the patient's phantasy of their omniscience and omnipotence, they might also believe that the patient has unconsciously caused what has happened. This phantasy may be a defense. This phantasy may be a defense against powerlessness for the therapist as well as the patient.

Lewis (1983) says a stillbirth is a "nothing baby." Where this baby should have been in the mother's mind, there is instead an autistic dead space. The Whites' denial of mourning for the dead infant also meant denial of the alive infant. The unconscious does not have "discrimination"—in the continuum of pregnancies and loss with the four miscarriages, the dead baby and the alive one were all experienced as one and the same. In the unconscious, there is no sense of time, no sense of space, and no separation of inner and outer reality. They saw the inner reality of their own deadness as being true of their external alive baby. Their dead external world was given a false life as they concentrated on the management of their milk run, but their alive inside world was deadened and the alive baby was also dead to them.

What unconscious logic allowed these parents to deny the existence of their twins, and even more that one was dead and one was alive, such that they could not "find time" to come in and discuss their baby? When Mrs. White said, "I had nothing. I didn't have a baby at all," she defended with no experience of birth and hence no experience of death. Lewis and Bourne (1989) in drawing on Freud's (1957b) theory say that mourning of a perinatal death requires processing feelings and lost hopes so that memories of the dead baby eventually assume a healthy perspective. If this process fails, forgetting becomes a desperate blocking out, a no-go area, and remembering becomes a haunted state of mind.

Denial has no memory. Memory can be shared and cried over. It was the team's allowing an experience of mourning, a finding of a dead baby, that allowed a finding of an alive one for Mr. and Mrs. White. In the resolution, the parents' despair and loss were validated, and the power of their denial was confronted. In acknowledging a dead infant, they could risk believing in an alive one. The team worked together respecting each other's role and the parents' rightful place. On revisits to the clinic Mr. and Mrs. White seemed absorbed in their baby. Each subsequent pregnancy may have taken away the opportunity to mourn the previous one (Lewis and Casement 1986). Lewis says that birth and death are perhaps impossible to think about, which is why stillbirth and death in pregnancy is so hard to cope with. Rayner (1981) says the conscious mind cannot cope with alive and dead in the same thought.

This was all too obvious in the case of Mr. and Mrs. White. The confusion was between being the victims, leaving them at the mercy of an external predator, or being the predators, leaving them terrified of their own capacity to destroy. There is either an unreal submission, or a plea entered into of their murderousness and hence massive guilt. The person in unresolved trauma cannot occupy their own central stage to balance these primitive aspects of their personality. Hence there is left an unoccupied center—an empty stage. Lewis and Casement (1986) showed how a pregnancy inhibits the process of mourning.

The alive presence of a container allows mourning to take place. The follow-up (after therapy) seems to show enough recovery for reasonable functioning. Immediate help given at the time of crisis is more timely and more beneficial than if dealt with years later. The deadening or autistic space is identifiable. It is the acknowledging of it that allows the experiencing of the psychic pain and the resolution. There is a return of affect, although it is hard to assess how effectively and with how much residual damage to the personality,.

## THERAPEUTIC TECHNIQUES

Two factors are essential to the treatment of trauma—to acknowledge and experience the autistic deadened space, and to hold it, interpret it and wait in it.

Frances Tustin writes about this type of case: "Such a deadened psychic space can come into being in early infancy when processes of 'adhesive-at-oneness' between either of the parents and the child seem to be traumatically interrupted when unexpected and painful awareness of their bodily separateness from each other is forced upon them. This assault occurs in a state which is beyond the infant's capacity to bear the pain of the trauma, so process it, and to come to terms with it . . . such children are 'numb and dumb'" (Tustin 1994, 117). They have been stunned and stunted by the trauma. The sudden awareness of their bodily separateness from a suckling mother's body with which they had felt everlastingly and erotically "at one," means that the nipple of the breast, or its substitute, is felt to be wrenched away from their mouth in a traumatically raping way (Tustin 1972). This pain spreads to other bodily orifices. Tracey tells us that in a psychic space of traumatized patients everything has come to a "dead stop." Lewis (1983) calls it a "no-go area." It is an "opting-out" area with suicide lurking in the wings. It is a deeply hidden split-off part that has "dropped out" of life and living because, at one time, life had been too painful for them. Avoiding the pain had enabled them to go on with life and living, but this had been at the cost of sacrificing originality and creativity. It is difficult for the analyst to get in touch with this deadened psychic space, especially in adult neurotic patients, because they will have become very adept at fending off attempts to do so. Also, it cannot be fully broached until the patient's internal structure is ready to cope with it.

The way that such traumatic psychic events can be affected therapeutically is by re-experiencing them in the "here and now" of the analysis. Originally, the traumatic experiences were wordless. Words in the form of interpretations and admonitions, though not unhelpful, will not be effective in the end. To be worked through, such a patient has to experience the suffering supported by internalized experiences with the analyst. Such an analysis requires great courage on the part of the analyst, and great trust in the patient. Those who experience such an analysis are indeed privileged.

## ACKNOWLEDGMENTS

My thanks to those who worked at the Royal Alexandra Children's Hospital, Camperdown on the case presented in this chapter. Helen Hardy was the occupational therapist; Barry Wythe was the pediatrician.

Norma Tracey (1991) "The Psychic Space in Trauma," Journal of Child Psychotherapy, 17 (2): 29–43., copyright © Association of Child Psychotherapists, reprinted by permission of Taylor & Francis Ltd, http://www.tandfonline.com on behalf of Association of Child Psychotherapists.

"Autistic Children who are Assessed as not Brain-damaged," Norma Tracey, Journal of Child Psychotherapy, 20 (1): 103–31., copyright © Association of Child Psychotherapists, reprinted by permission of Taylor & Francis Ltd, http://www.tandfonline.com on behalf of Association of Child Psychotherapists.

# *Chapter 6*

# Working With Depressed Mothers in the Early Months of Their Infant's Life

This chapter illustrates how my work has developed over the years and informed my thinking about, and work with, depressed mothers. It draws on a central theme: the depressed mother, returning to her own infant beginnings through pregnancy and birth, confronts a dead mother–dead infant dyad. Trauma from the mother's own infancy is seen to have created an internal, autistic, deadened psychic space. It is argued that behind this deadness lies the primal pain of abandonment and loss. The associated rage, previously repressed but now awakened by her alive infant and its powerful primitive demands, invade the mother's psyche. The internal deadness freezes her alive processes as mother to her baby. Unbearable pain is awakened, and she may be in terror and unable to move, or she may experience herself as drowning in something catastrophic.

## BACKGROUND

As a social worker in a children's hospital many years ago, I often saw mothers sitting by their sick infant's bed with a far-off "autistic-like" vacant look, as if they were not there. In interviews with these mothers, I was always aware that, even if they appeared animated, there was an unreal, cut-off quality to their narrative, as if they were speaking about someone else and were not there with you. I wrote at the time that these mothers were traumatized by their child's illness and that central to their trauma was fear of death. I wrote of an autistic core space created by this trauma: "There is unthinkable fear, so there is no thinking . . . what is left is non-living space, where knowing would be if it could be known, where thinking would be if it could be thought. This space has an autistic, deadening quality. Its cause is demonstrably similar to that described by Tustin (1972) in autistic children" (Tracey 1991, 29). I argued that recovery for these mothers was not a return to their previous pattern of thinking and being, but rather, there was a period of disturbance and considerable suffering. I suggested that the trauma, which could not initially be dealt with and had been repressed in its raw primitive state, was now exposed and that the dosage and the timing in terms of the capacity to "suffer" the suffering was all too relevant (Tracey 1991, 37). I had taken Frances Tustin's concept of autism in infancy and shown how adult responses during trauma appeared to be similar. Tustin, on reading my paper, began a correspondence that continued up till her death. In one of her articles she wrote, "I have quoted extensively from Norma Tracey's paper, because it says so much of what I have found to be true, and also adds to my understanding" (Tustin 1994, 117)

Although she felt she was too old to share in my subsequent work, she directed, encouraged, and inspired me to undertake it. This was research with mothers and fathers of premature infants (Tracey 2000). The mothers presented as emotionally numbed, unable to think or process. They did not register overt depression in the same way as the mothers of normal infants, just a "flatness"—no emotion at all. In our professional group, we could see clearly how the mother's numbness later led to a very disturbed state, in which her inner world was enacted with the people around her without discernment or judgment, and created havoc (Tracey et al. 1995, 47). Now that the danger of death had passed, they were free to experience the emotions and fear associated with the possible loss of their infant and, in some cases, fear of their own death. We hypothesized was that behind the deadness lay a primitive passionate aliveness too catastrophic to be experienced. The primitive nature of the paranoid fear affected anyone who listened to the tapes of the research interviews, particularly the two colleagues who did the rating (Garner 2000).

After this research, I undertook a preliminary study of women who were depressed in the first year of their baby's life. It seemed like an obvious next step to take. In many cases, these women had healthy full-term infants, normal birth, and often a satisfactory family and social life, but their emotions did not seem very different from those of the traumatized mothers of premature babies. They appeared to have been affected most severely by the normal birth processes of ordinary motherhood. They seemed to be in the same autistic-like space, often followed by primitive emotions and disturbed and sometimes disturbing behavior. Working with groups of pregnant women and women with newborn babies, I began to formulate the idea that, since trauma resided in such a sensory, physical and primitive area of our being, the primitive and physical event of birth could in itself unleash previous infantile, childhood or adolescent traumas, which also reside in that same sensory, physical and primitive area. This is described by Bion (1962, 1963) in psychodynamic terms (beta elements), and by van der Kolk et al. (1996, 85) in physiological terms. In psychodynamic terms, during pregnancy or in giving birth, women return to their own infancy and primeval mother (Pines 1972; Green 1986; Hedges 1994). This understanding led us to speculate as to how the infant in the mind of the mother became deadened. How did this state of affairs come about?

## THEORETICAL CONSTRUCTS IN THINKING ABOUT DEPRESSED MOTHERS

The depressed mother, it seems to me, has lost her central core of identity. She seems not to have a meaning or value for herself as a mother to her infant; she seems to be in mourning, as if she had suffered a terrible loss. One has no sense of her being protected by internal "good" objects. It is as if the "good" internal mother has died and is lost to her, and she is left at the mercy of internal persecutory destructive forces. Some of the elements of behavior and thought could be described as paranoid and psychotic, but uppermost is a sense of terror, as if death is too close or has already occurred. The mother's discrimination of unconscious and conscious is lost. Projections go from person to person without real discrimination. Time seems lost, and old hurts become confused with present ones. There is a shattering of the belief that things can go right for her or that she has a right to expect that they will. There is a sense of being "cursed" rather than blessed, of being punished rather than rewarded.

What does all this signify? These symptoms are very similar to those of mothers whose infants are ill or dying. It seems that the psychic pain caused by chaos and by the loss of the old identity as she moves toward her new identity as a mother is intolerable. Bion (1957) first gave us the idea of psychotic and nonpsychotic twin elements of self, surviving side by side. Sydney Klein (1981, 103) developed Bion's idea further in his paper "Autistic Phenomena in Neurotic Patients." He suggested that the psychotic twin in adults may be an autistic psychotic infant residing in a normal adult due to a catastrophe in infancy. Sydney Klein's ideas may serve as pointers toward understanding the depressed mother who, in having her external healthy infant, may in fact also be opening the door to her dead infant–dead mother psychotic dyad.

Green (1986) speaks of the "dead mother" as a mother who is known through sensual pleasure and then, when she fails to appear when needed, becomes internalized as lost and dead. Green holds that the dead mother remains as a blank or dead space in our psyche, an area where love and desire once held life and potential. I want to take this proposition further and suggest that behind this deadened mother—this empty psychic stage—are characters with paranoid, angry, primitive emotions born out of unrequited needs. The murderous rage of frustration creates a catastrophe the infant cannot cope with. The terror is too much. The infant closes down. The infant and the mother of the infant die to each other. While there is death and the repression of these feelings, the mother does not hear the "loud noise" of her primeval desires but when there is a real, alive baby with just such primitive needs and desires, the terror and the intolerable suffering are awakened once more. There is terror is at the center of the shutdown, although a death-like shutdown in itself is a mechanism to avoid the catastrophe of death and disintegration. The depressed mother therefore often has a terror of human contact, even fearing to leave the house. The terror is that if she "comes to life" she will bring her infant death rather than life, harm rather than good. This psychotic or disorganized "pocket" inside her psyche might never have been exposed had she not become pregnant. Many women may even get pregnant in the hope of finding the alive mother and the alive baby through an alive infant and mother outside. This gives some understanding of the resistance of a depressed mother to experiencing or rather re-experiencing this intense primordial psychic agony of loss and abandonment. For the depressed mother the "holding," "at one with," "containing" mother is dead and absent. What is relevant is that the birth of her infant has awakened her awareness of death within. The shock, the terror of death central to the ordeal, becomes beyond a mother's emotional endurance yet again.

## CATASTROPHE AND FAITH

The depressed mother is unable to access the "area of faith." Eigen's work provides a particularly useful way of formulating a kind of construct as to what might be happening for the depressed mother. Identifying a difference between Melanie Klein and Wilfred Bion, he writes, "Both Klein and Winnicott saturated the arrival at the depressive position with a kind of 'moral' goodness, but the value of paranoia was ignored or passed over. [However,] Bion saw the paranoid and the depressive position as mutually dependent. Bion saw daring to enter catastrophe to disintegrate, to break apart, as the psychic event that gives birth to new thinking" Eigen (1985, 325).

Bion sees it as an innate part of the self's rhythm to fall apart and to come together again. Out of this perception, I conceive that the problem of the depressed mother is that she has no faith that if she falls apart, she will come together again; indeed, she has proof in her past of being unheld and of not coming together again. She is frozen in terror and dares not to go into catastrophe, so there is no resolution, no arrival at her own identity. She is left at the mercy of raw unprocessed emotions, which Bion (1963, 99) describes as beta elements, "a mixed state in which the patient is persecuted by feelings of depression and depressed by feelings of persecution." This, he says, all points to catastrophe. I would suggest that, at some early stage in the depressed mother's life, the "holder of the faith," her mother, has failed her and has failed to hold her through the catastrophe. The catastrophe, being in consequence too much to tolerate, has caused disassociation and deadness. The movement between faith and catastrophe is frozen. The problem of the depressed mother is that she dare not go mad and therefore cannot reach sanity. She has lost faith. The place where faith and catastrophe meet, where self is born, where knowing can occur, is not accessible to her. This hypothesis corresponds with Tustin's work on psychological birth and psychological catastrophe. She writes of a premature rupturing of the "at-oneness" of mother and infant due to the mother's failure to be there for the infant (Tustin 1981, 181).

The following material from a depressed mother illustrates and gives reality to this area of catastrophe and faith: "I often wonder how I've survived so long without going crazy or having a nervous breakdown. I worry that any day I will just collapse in a heap or go off the deep end. I feel like I'm on the edge of disaster." This sense of "on the edge of disaster" is an oft-repeated theme. The concern here is that catastrophe will take over and the return to normal thinking or judgment will be lost to her. This is the loss of the area of faith. The loss of faith and the fear of going into catastrophe and not being able to survive it can be seen from this next quote:

> I feel sick with all the emotions, I feel so desperate. These feelings scare me. I remember so clearly the night I couldn't control my tears and emotions—I was totally out of control and became more and more hysterical. I could see Phillip trying to cope with the situation as best he could. After crying in bed for about an hour he got me up, we had tea, talked a little and an hour or so later we went to bed exhausted. It worries me that it might happen again; I don't want that because it was a horrible experience. I'm here alone with Jonathon and I find myself holding back afraid of becoming hysterical and out of control. I feel so alone. (Except from research interview, 2004)

This is something like the "fear of breakdown," which Winnicott (1986) describes. This terror of being out of control is a terror of never gaining control again. The area of faith is lost.

## PSYCHOBIOLOGICAL BASIS

Research now compels us to view ourselves as an integrated physiological and psychological unit. The work of Perry et al. (1995) on the effects of trauma in infancy shows how the psychological results of trauma have biological antecedents; emotional neglect in infancy can cause major changes in the pathways of emotional response. Steffens et al. (1993) have described the physiological basis of depression and mania. The work of van der Kolk and Saporta (1993) illustrates the physiological basis for the symptoms we see in trauma and the consequent numbing. It may be therefore that psychobiological events in the mother's infancy have caused the depression to present itself now in motherhood.

> Children and infants use a variety of adaptive response patterns in the face of threat, and, in use-dependent fashion, internalize aspects of these responses, organizing the developing brain. (Perry et al. 1995, 286)

> Hundreds of animal studies . . . [show] that a narrow window—a critical period—exists during which specific sensory experience is required for optimal organization and development of the part of the brain mediating a specific function. (Perry et al. 1995, 276)

Perry et al. note that infantile or childhood trauma can lead to complex character adaptations and disturbed regulation of affective arousal. Dissociation, somatization and affect dysregulation are seen as the results of this disturbance. I suggest, as Perry et al. do, that the infant's vulnerability gives any negative experience a lasting effect both physically and psychically. I would add to this that trauma, whether singular or accumulated, can create areas or pockets of autism, can be dissociated and repressed and then reawakened through the psychophysical events of pregnancy and birth. If such trauma, or accumulated trauma, occur in the sensitive time of infancy, could the physical experience of birth and the physical vulnerability of this time awaken memories stored not in the mind but as bodily sensations, memories akin to terror of death and catastrophe? This would fit the thinking of van der Kolk and Saporta (1993), who see terror of death as central to all traumas, and of Bion (1963), who identifies the beta elements as pointing to catastrophe.

### Numbing

The "numbing" caused by trauma, the emotions of the event remaining unable to be processed and in their raw state, is well documented by many authors, including Bion (1963), Klein (1981), Tustin (1994) and Tracey

(2000). Now, as a result of van der Kolk and Saporta's work (1993), numbing is recognized as having a physiological basis as part of the response to trauma. They found that twenty years after the original trauma, people with post-traumatic stress disorder developed opioid-mediated analgesia in response to a stimulant resembling the traumatic stressor. Just as there is a physiological basis to depression, so too we have a physiological basis for the repression and numbing that leads to the formation of an autistic core. This raises the question of what factors in the mother's infancy could have caused this, and how did it happen?

## THE UNMET NEEDS OF A MOTHER AS AN INFANT

There is a plethora of literature that demonstrates the need for a caring and responsive parent and the serious results of an absent or emotionally absent parent, and how such events in childhood inform and create the depressed mother. Spitz's (1945) seminal paper on "hospitalism" brought to our attention the effect on infants left with inadequate mothering. Hospitalism, as defined by Spitz (1945, 53), "designates a vitiated condition of the body due to long confinement in hospital, or the morbid condition of the atmosphere of the hospital. The term has been increasingly preempted to specify the evil effect of institutional care on infants placed in institutions from an early age, particularly from the psychiatric point of view." The mother's psychic care-taking and emotional presence were absent or limited for the infants in Spitz's study and the results were quite serious disturbances and possible morbidity. "There is a point under which the mother-child relations cannot be restricted during the child's first year without irreparable damage," Spitz (1945) writes. I suggest that if the infant suffered deprivation of a more limited nature, the results could be pockets of deadness, not in the body but in the psyche.

Bowlby (1969, 1973), in his work on attachment and loss, defined the stages of an infant or child's emotional response to a physically absent mother: the movement from crying out in need, the cries becoming more desperate, the stage of severe protest, and then the infant giving up and becoming "autistic-like." Bowlby's description is not very different from that described by van der Kolk in post-traumatic stress, and it seems to fit the autistic pocket of which I write.

Bowlby's work inspired a number of other studies, begun by Ainsworth et al. (1978). Ainsworth's research, and that of others, shows that the type of attachment between mother and infant has a very significant effect on the infant's emotional life. The importance of attunement has been another important area of research. Tronick and Cohn (1988) note that the mother–infant dyad sends out thousands of invisible tendrils, reaching and searching for how each can find a response that can best connect to the other. They report that attempts to connect succeed in only 30 percent of cases. How does it happen that loving human extension is not met and therefore allowed to wither and die? What is the nature of the internalized experience of the infant when he reaches out and this call is unmet? It is proposed that a record of frustration, loss or disappointment is imprinted on that infant's unconscious psyche. The turning away of the infant, seeking self-comforting and "cutting off" in Tronick and Cohn's still-face experiments, gives evidence of this (Cohn and Tronick, 1983; Tronick et al., 1982). Tronick and Cohn (1988) provide further evidence of negative affect and disrupted behavior in the infant if the mother is not responsive. The work of Trevarthen (1980) and Stern (1985, 1995) shows that infants' innate ability to differentiate and use affective information in the facial and bodily cues of familiar caregivers is an important prerequisite for regulating their own emotions and responses.

The studies, whether from attachment research or the psychodynamic, ego- or self-psychology schools, all agree on this one point. The mother's capacity to be in tune with her infant is all-important for the infant's psychic survival. Fonagy et al. (1992) confirmed Selma Fraiberg's observations concerning the re-emergence of childhood conflicts at early stages of child rearing. They saw the mother's capacity to reflect as dependent on her past relationships with key people in her life. The effect of the emotionally absent parent, who cannot link in with her infant's signals and desires because she is preoccupied, leaves the infant feeling meaningless and dead. I think that this is what has happened to the depressed mother, and it puts her in a position to repeat the cycle with her own infant. Failure to intervene is likely to perpetuate an intergenerational problem.

In his book, *In Search of the Lost Mother of Infancy*, Hedges (1994, 32) adds to this thesis the idea that "a living record of failed connection remains imprinted in our psyche" from our infancy. These imprints become the core or kernel of psychoses as enclaves, pockets or "layerings" of organizing processes in our infancy. Hedges believes the earliest lack of human contact to be so traumatizing that withdrawal occurs in the infant's psyche with far-reaching results into adult life. This withdrawal from the world of ordinary interpersonal relatedness is what I have described in the depressed mother. Hedges sees such people as having a terror of contact leading to a prevention of bonding. Extreme cases of depression in the mother appear to arise from trauma that occurred preverbally, very early in the infant's life. Further trauma at any stage of the human cycle may add to the effects of this, either because of the strength of the trauma or because of the sensitivity of the period, such as illness or the death of a partner during pregnancy.

The links with these traumas are relevant in understanding the depressed mother's misperception of her present live infant. Many women in pregnancy use their babies as a therapeutic object; their own needs and illusions become more important than the infant within. The interfering reality of the alive infant is threatening to the fixation to a "core relationship" to her own mother. As a result, her preoccupation with her infant is derailed; idealization and manic defense give way to disillusionment, rage, paranoid features, and severe depression. The idealization is a defense against deadness. The reality of the infant, his demandingness, his ruthless greed, his tyrannical rage, awaken aspects of her own murderousness and of her own murderous mother. Tischler (1979, 34) says, "The shadow of a mother's early 'bad,' 'destroyed' and punitive mother falls between her and her infant. Fantasies and images related to such a harsh, damaged internal mother and bad aspects of self, guilt feelings and the need for punishment invade her relationship with him and colour her illusions about him."

The infant's constancy as a good object is lost. In this way primary maternal preoccupation becomes contaminated by the mother's wishes for him to nurture her and meet her instincts and needs. When he fails to do this he is not protected from his own internal needs; there is no container, in Bion's sense, the mother is unable to receive and process his needs.

## CENTRAL THESIS

At the core of the mother's depression is either an internal dead mother and an internal dead baby, an internal destructive mother who kills babies, or an internal destructive infant who kills mothers. The depressed mother fears that death is more powerful than life; the destructive mother within is more powerful than the internal alive mother. The young mother, seeking out alive internal objects for her own nourishment and identity, is confronted by death and punishment and therefore inordinate guilt. She deadens her internal world, externally moves into a lifeless state, abdicates care of her infant and is haunted and tortured, or totally dependent and deadened. When she comes to life again, it is not a return to normality; the emotions, which previously could not be tolerated because of their primitive power, must now be experienced. The suffering and torment in this can be terrible, as described later. It is as if an internal wound, hidden and protected, is now opened and must be dealt with. It may be a temporary state easily dealt with; it may be all-pervading and require months or years of work; it may require psychotherapy, group therapy or family therapy; the mother may need medication; she may need hospitalization.

The eroding of her power as a woman and mother is central to this theme. The good-enough mother moves between a backward pull to passive being and a forward push to active becoming; she separates from her ideal inner mother to confront the terror of death from her inner destructive one; she wins through to become an alive mother to her infant. This triumph over death is her center of power. This allows the emergence of a powerful new mediating center. The depressed mother does not find her center of power. This is tragic, because it is from this center of power that she is the provider and protector of her infant's needs. The sense of weakness and powerlessness is one of the primary symptoms we all know well in the depressed mother. All the joy that comes from being a life-giving mother; the feeling of being at the center of creativity; the privacy of the enclosed circle between mother and infant; all these are intruded on. She feels ever at war in a battle she cannot win, or that she has already lost.

In postnatal depression, mourning becomes melancholia. The woman mourns not just a loss of the infant from her womb but also the loss of "her own mother" who has died inside her infant self in the past. She does not find the alive mother again. She now feels she has an internal dead mother and experiences herself as dead. What she has is a "no-go" area of primitive destruction, and covering this there is a non-thinking space because the thoughts are too terrible to be thought. No reflection or reverie can take place; she cannot see or hear her infant. Melanie Klein (1946) described the dynamic of the constant struggle between an irrepressible urge to destroy one's objects and the desire to preserve them. My supposition is that the depressed mother does not believe that her "life-giving" capacity is as great as her capacity to destroy. Such a fantasy is terrifying to the mother. She fears her own destructiveness will make the infant ill or will come from a destructive mother within herself as a punishment for her sexuality or rivalry with her mother.

Sometimes a mother of a newborn may have a dream of having the Christ child, the Messiah, which is replaced by the reality of a helpless, vulnerable infant. She needs to surrender the dream and accept the reality. There is the complete relief that the baby is not damaged, but is a quite ordinary human being. The depressed mother may feel that: (a) in losing the dream, she has totally lost the real baby; (b) she has the real baby but is undeserving of her baby because of guilt feelings of rivalry with her mother; or (c) in separating out from her own mother she will go mad. Any of these three factors will intrude on the negotiating processes between the mother and her baby. The surrender of the dream and attachment to the real infant is a process that goes on between a mother and an infant. In every negotiated moment with the baby she gives up a bit of the dream and she settles for the reality of her infant and the reality of herself as mother.

Confronted with this internal drama, there is a well-defined role for the worker. By her empathic presence, she provides an immutable holding space where the drama can unfreeze and where she can be an alive "mother" to the mother. Some of the case material presented below highlights the difficulties in treating the depressed mother and the deadness and the autistic core I have described.

## CASE 1: ANNA

Anna had a traumatic birth with her very premature baby, in which there was a risk of death to herself and her infant. Anna's mother committed suicide five years before the birth of this baby. All nine interviews with Anna were audiotaped and the material from these interviews is used with her permission. This is a direct quote from the audiotape:

> I'm so afraid of getting her home. She will go off her brain because babies sometimes go off their brains. Oh God! I'm getting sweaty palms now just thinking of it. OK, so I might as well tell you about these angry feelings that well up in me. I know they are good feelings to have after what I've been through, they are just part of living like burping and farting and breathing. I didn't realize until today, my God I'm 37, and my mother keeps coming back to me, it's not she couldn't handle my feelings of anger, she couldn't handle her own feelings of anger, and I'm scared when I see this little thing go off her brain, I can't cope because it is going to bring up all my own stuff, and I've got to lock it away so I don't see it. I'm angry with my father too, why didn't he rip his shirt off and show the superman's insignia underneath and come in. I'm even more scared because I'm not a baby sort of person. You know how some people go "goo-goo!" I'm not like that.

Highlighted in this account by a depressed mother is the fear of her own destructiveness. There is also a fear of going mad or having a mad infant. With that part of herself that does not go "goo-goo" to her baby, she seemed to be describing the dead, nonresponsive mother inside her. Over the nine interviews I had with Anna, this unreal kind of response was very evident. Like so many of the other mothers, Anna would laugh inappropriately at terrible things and, in the middle of the interview, her voice would change and she would say, "There, there Anna! We must pull ourselves together!" and give herself a slap on the wrist. This I came to understand as her desperate effort to keep herself alive with her dead mother inside her. Anna enacted an alive mother to herself, but it had a strange feeling about it, as if it were a caricature. Anna became more anxious on taking her baby home. She became terrified of lead in the soil and covered all the windows with sheets to keep the lead out. She could not go to the toilet without taking the baby with her. Sometimes laughing, mocking and manic, I actually felt Anna was more real when she could speak of her fears, as in the quote above from the sixth interview. She would then speak more in a sad, settled manner. When the baby was aged three months, Anna became too depressed to stay with her and decided in a manic way to return to part-time work, saying that it would keep her sane and she would be better for her baby if she remained sane. (Anna is a health professional. No one is immune.)

## CASE 2: VIVIENNE

Vivienne is the mother of a healthy full-term infant, referred by an infant health center for a postnatal depression study. In her contact telephone call she said, "I have postnatal depression. I really need help." The following material is transcribed directly from the audiotape, but for reasons of brevity it has been edited here:

> Can I start from the beginning? OK, this is my first baby, a little girl, Marietta, born in May this year. I was disgustingly healthy, and everything ran smoothly through the pregnancy. So I had Marietta in May and everything about the birth was fine, and she was a perfect healthy little girl. Exactly two weeks after Marietta was born I had a very bad postpartum secondary hemorrhage and I was rushed to hospital. I was all right that morning, but by lunchtime I was feeling really ill. Phillip went to golf. I was so distressed at being abandoned by him. I could not believe he would go and leave me with a new baby and sick and go out like that. I was in tears the whole afternoon. He came home early cause it was raining. I began to bleed so profusely I was terrified; I did not know what was going on. When he came in, it looked like a massacre had happened. We rang the hospital straightaway and the midwife said, "Pack a bag and come in." I was nearly unconscious.
>
> I had a very nasty experience with the doctor at the hospital, and that left a very sour taste in my mouth. He basically walked in, told me who he was, didn't tell me what he was going to do. He inserted a speculum, and he broke all my stitches. I was screaming. Then basically he left just saying, "No! We have to get her to surgery." I had emergency surgery. They did a D&C [dilation and curettage]. I couldn't even sit up without fainting.
>
> This particular doctor came to me the very next day, which was about 10 hours after the surgery, and told me I could go home. I couldn't even sit up without fainting, that's how bad I was. So of course the nurses got very concerned. Towards the end of the day I was getting worse. They rang my obstetrician and as a result I was kept in and two IVs were put into my arm. My own obstetrician was so good and was horrified at how the other one had treated me. And so that was that drama.

This basic splitting of one good and one bad person may well have been true in reality, but it is present in every depressed mother I see. The other important point to note is the dull matter-of-fact voice in which all of this is related. Medical terms such as "antibiotics" and "hemoglobin" would have been foreign to this mother but, as is often the case, they are held on to as if to create some sense of control in an uncontrollable situation. Vivienne could have been talking about someone else, and I felt throughout the interview that there was an overly animated "story" but that she was not in it. I had no feeling of being invited to be aware of her feelings.

> So I came home, I had probably a hemoglobin level of about five or six so I wasn't able to function very well at home. So I went to live with my mother for a while. So immediately the family is dysfunctional, OK! Phillip is away from the baby and me. I couldn't take care of the baby; the baby was taken straight to my mother's place, where she looked after her while I was in hospital. I couldn't breastfeed because all the antibiotics that were going through my milk were upsetting the baby terribly so that was very distressing. Then my doctor told me to keep pumping as in expressing, so I pumped for over a month to try and keep my milk going and then I was told that I wasn't allowed to breastfeed any longer because I was too weak and too anemic and too run down.

Here is more of the confusion I am accustomed to seeing in the depressed mother. She is talking about the husband's absence, the baby being taken from her, her milk drying up, her family lost to her—loss upon loss. Everywhere is chaos and confusion, but all related like some interesting story.

> When I finally went home, I was so tired I couldn't enjoy my little baby. So my husband did help me through a lot of the night feeds at that time. Looking back and on reflection I was a complete zombie, I just could not function. I was feeling so dreadful in myself because motherhood, everything that I thought motherhood was going to be wasn't. My husband is a company director and he works from 7.30 in the morning till about 7 o'clock at night, so I was left on my own.

The description of being zombie-like, taking no joy in the baby, exhausted, unable to function, being on her own and unsupported is a common one, but unusually did not elicit a feeling of empathy in me.

> So the baby had been unsettled as well. Anyway, so I started to feel really sick in myself, and I started to feel like I was getting even more run down, and the doctors kept saying to me it's just because you've lost so much blood, and so Dr. Jones organized for myself and the baby to go to Tresillian [a nursing care institution for mothers having difficulties with babies]. They took me in a second and I went there really for my sake, just to have a rest. I started to worry about going home. I knew my husband would neglect me; I started to bleed

again. They rushed me off to the doctor who was just down the road and he diagnosed me as having chronic fatigue, and they encouraged me to stay another week which I did.

As soon as I got home, I started to feel really low in myself and I wasn't coping during the day. My marriage was falling apart; we were arguing all the time, my husband couldn't work out why I was so stressed and wasn't coping. It placed unbelievable strain on our relationship because I was giving so much to the baby during the day that by the time he got home from work I had nothing else to give. I was basically just existing. I felt dead on the inside, and when I started to feel anything, I had all these terrible negative feelings going around on the inside. I felt ripped off because I had been so sick in the four months of Marietta's life that I hadn't been able to enjoy her or motherhood. It was nothing like I thought it was going to be. And of course, as time went on and my marriage seemed to be getting worse, I felt totally isolated at home. I didn't want to talk to anybody, I couldn't communicate with him, because he didn't seem to understand. There was a point there when he was saying, "You know I'm sick of you being sick, what's the matter with you? Why are you feeling this way, you know you're always sour, you're always unhappy, you should be the happiest girl in the world? You've got a wonderful little baby girl."

I felt very ashamed because I've always been such a strong girl and then for this to happen. It was out of my control, I couldn't control how I was feeling, I couldn't control what was happening to my marriage. I felt like I couldn't be a good mother to Marietta because I couldn't enjoy it. I had no energy to do anything else. I would cook dinner during the day when Marietta was napping so that I could then rest and all I would have to do is just reheat it and then I could go to bed. In those days I was going to bed at 7.30, 8 o'clock. I'm sure my husband has his own feelings of being totally rejected but it's difficult for me given that I have had such a life of being around so many people [she is an international air hostess], then to be totally isolated at home, with a baby, and feeling so sick and then of course discovering that I had postnatal depression. I'd say this has been the worst five months of my whole life. All the thoughts about my father's neglect of me came to the fore, and I could see I married a man just like him. Worst of all was the thought that I was becoming weak like my mother. She is a nothing to my dominating bullying father.

Vivienne continued in a similar vein, not pausing for breath, and at the end said, "There is the story, now you have it." As a therapist I had sat through what should have been a harrowing story with no feeling whatever, and very few thoughts. Nevertheless, she seemed keen to return and I made another appointment.

What happened then amazed me. As she was leaving it seemed as if the real depression became exposed. I'm sure she experienced it also. I was overwhelmed. The unrelieved blackness seemed directly linked with separating, leaving the session, communicated by very forceful projective identification.

The therapy became alive, but this was characterized by constant acting out. She never paid a bill. She often did not come for the most trivial reasons, like having also booked a hairdressing appointment. She resented immensely that she should have to pay. It was my duty to treat her. Her treatment of her husband, in the joint sessions I had with them, was worse than anything she dealt out to me. She broke off therapy and they separated. She phoned, crying like a child, asking me to see her again. They came back together. After a session where she cried because I discussed the fee, and she complained about her impoverishment, she rang me a day later to say she was flying to New Zealand to visit a lovely aunt who would look after her. Her husband pleaded that he was being deprived of his baby. She returned, and then moved in with her parents and he had to phone to ask permission to see his infant—permission they often did not give. He entered therapy in his own right, and she would ring me like a child asking me to see her, but as soon as I agreed she was even more arrogantly scathing. Later she could not find the time for me as she returned to her glamorous job and her mother, in a martyred way, looked after the baby full time.

Did I help in any way? My discussion group kept encouraging me to keep seeing her. I did not understand why. I felt unwilling, consigned to a role in a drama I had not created, in which I did not really belong and over which I had no control. The literature about the depressed woman in the postnatal phase seems not to refer to the degree of hatred these women suffer, sometimes towards themselves, sometimes towards their partner. The transference is often powerfully hateful. The "as if "seems to be gone; the rage over the need to ask for help, over having to pay for it, is enormous. Have they already paid the dead mother too much and feel they owe no more? There is murder and death and unfair judgment in the air and it is hard to tell who has done what to whom.

In Vivienne's case I would suggest that there was a dead internal mother, and that Vivienne was terrified of her infant killing her, by restricting her and keeping her at home. In later sessions she told me that her own mother was extremely depressed and had once needed hospitalization. Vivienne spent a session talking about her father's dominance and control during her early childhood and even in adult life. He had crushed her mother. Vivienne had escaped into her glamorous profession so as never to be like her mother and never to be controlled. Motherhood threatened her in every way. I always felt that she used me as a kind of lowly servant. This was interesting because this is what she also did to her mother, as her mother became the permanent nanny. This must be what she thought motherhood was—a depressed and lowly state. Motherhood threatened the manic false self with the possibility of a real self, but this real self, meant awakening from the internal deadness and coping with real depression, the depression that she and I had jointly experienced at the end of the first session. Vivienne's profession was well suited as a manic escape, and she would have coped well had she not become pregnant and had an infant, opening all the areas within that had not been dealt with.

There is a need to be able to use a holding space. Many mothers are not motivated enough to allow such holding. They are desperate for symptomatic relief only. Others use it as an opportunity to work through serious inner difficulties, to get things right for themselves. Many oedipal factors come to life in an extraordinarily real way, and previously unresolved conflicts to do with love, hate or envy present themselves at this vulnerable time. The idealization of motherhood as beautiful and caring is often a defense against facing the power of the mother to frustrate the child and refuse love to her, load her with guilt, or make her feel bad for just being. When she comes, in turn, to give birth and is hurled back to her own earliest beginnings, she may hate the mother she has become; she may be caught in the envy of her own mother; or, in the ambivalence of love and hate, she may feel guilt and anxiety. As Main (1968, 159) puts it, "Maternity tests the whole system of the early hidden rivalries and guilt of the Oedipus situation and of the mental defenses against these. Maternity, the final sexual achievement of the girl, therefore, carries with it the greatest potential for arousing the hatred of the internalized Oedipal mother-rivalry and for producing a sense of crushing guilt and anxiety."

The depressed mothers I see teach me a great deal about the incredible depth of emotions exposed by motherhood; and about not necessarily being able to conduct therapy within the session-room structure, when the depressed mother is functioning at such a primitive level. Some mothers leave, as Vivienne did, with no sense of resolution, but I could understand what she was escaping from as she left me to carry the depression and anxiety of abandonment. I felt useless and helpless, deadened, very like the dead mother who may be inside her. Often the depressed mother is looking for relief from this sense of deadness or from the primitive emotions behind the deadness that reveal, as with Vivienne, unbelievable suffering, but this is not necessarily the same as wanting therapy; this makes the treatment of such mothers harder. Therapy requires the capacity to survive and suffer what has previously been insufferable.

In Winnicott's classic paper, "Fear of Breakdown" (1986), he wrote of patients who have a terror of a future catastrophe: "I feel like I'm on the edge of disaster." Winnicott described how the catastrophe had already occurred in the past. This fits the model I am describing. For these depressed mothers, the raw terror of a previous breakdown is perceived as a breakdown to come. Their inner world is made up of horrific actors unable to be allowed to perform on their life stage because they are so terrible. The empty stage or space is autistic-like. These mothers appear vacant and dead, at the mercy of the internal deadly mother of their infancy who "kills" by being unavailable. Often, such a negative transference is projected onto the therapist, who is seen as the original deadly mother, and the patient experiences herself as pathologically infantilized and motherless. Working with these mothers is not always successful and sometimes the neutral analytic stance can feel to be not unlike the internal dead mother. I have found one way to handle this is to be more actively and "holdingly" interpretative. I have not always been successful.

Many depressed mothers feel that the only way they can placate the monstrous mother within is by stripping themselves of the joy of mothering. They mold it into a punitive experience, deny their fault in it and see their partner as to blame, or carry the entire fault and become crippled with guilt, feeling they have robbed their own mother of life by being alive. The problems of sexual enjoyment after giving birth occur not only because of the pain and the physical experiences involved but also because of the unconscious guilt and fear of enjoying one's body again. Even more extreme than this, in some women guilt about genital activity is savagely severe, too great to be atoned for by mere suffering. The clinical state of such women is one of helpless suffering and depression which takes many forms, but in which some features are constant. Far from enjoying her baby, the mother is afraid of him, averse to him, or apathetic about him. She is unable to own him fully and fiercely as her own, and she may feel that he is not really hers. Ill-equipped for motherhood, she feeds or attends the baby too little or too much, too rarely or too often, and is envious of the better care anyone else would be able to give her baby. Cooking, cleaning, and other wifely or maternal functions are not now pleasurable but exhausting, to be undertaken with suffering and anxiety. Sexual life with her husband is painful, her husband is seen as intolerable and selfish in his wishes for pleasure, and there are quarrels. The guilt about having the child is in this way paid for by renouncing joys. She may retreat from adult life with its forbidden pleasures and its guilt-laden conflicts into a state of anxious, childlike helplessness, running back to her mother.

## CASE 3: JULIANNE

Julianne, a highly intelligent lawyer, attended one of our mothers' groups where her strange, switched-off, autistic-like manner could be seen. She attended all the groups but seemed never to be present, often leaving in the middle of a group or three-quarters of the way through to take her infant home, but never saying "goodbye." She later told me she spent days on her own in her sixth-floor unit, feeling that the only way to end her misery would be to kill herself and her baby, or have the baby adopted by someone more deserving of an infant. She hid these thoughts from her husband and from all in our group, as daily they began to take over more and more of her mind. This reached a peak in somatization. She developed severe back pain. She told us this was from the weight of her baby when she carried him. Thoughts had come to my mind of a "dead" weight and of her as a "dead" mother. Julianne asked her mother whether she would mind Tom, the baby, while Julianne went to the chiropractor. The mother arrived to do this, and Julianne told us what happened.

> She walked into the baby's room, and I was in chaos. I couldn't think to find anything. My mother, who had never minded Tom before, said, "I knew it would come to this; I've missed my bridge day, I told you not to have children, you're the brainy type; I knew you couldn't cope with motherhood." The terrible pain of my back and such prophetic remarks now hurt beyond anything I could endure. I screamed back at her, "You've never seen me as a person, just a brain!."

Julianne is a monotonal, quiet person and I found it hard to even imagine her screaming. Julianne then recounted that her mother said, "I'm not going to be talked to like that," and stormed out. Julianne was left alone with her aching back and her crying baby and no appointment with the chiropractor. After a sleepless night, Julianne decided to face her mother. When she went to the house her mother opened the door and said, "Who are you?" and closed it in her face. I wondered if she could not cope with her daughter coming "alive," and did not know her. That day in the group, Julianne sobbed as she told the story to us. Everyone in the room was aghast. We had never seen Julianne cry. Other mothers started to cry, as if in sympathy for her, but some also remembering problems between themselves and their mothers.

They began talking. "I've got nothing on today, I'll stay with her now and this afternoon." "I can come tomorrow," another said. "We could go walking on Friday," another offered. The mothers kept up the visiting, going for walks and having coffee together. About four weeks later, Julianne arrived at the group. "Hey, everyone! I've baked a cake. My first cake ever, you understand, ever." Everyone must have understood what it meant because they applauded. I felt the cake was a symbol of her believing in herself as a mother, organizing to collect the ingredients and then producing something good and alive like a freshly baked cake. The depressed mother is often unable to organize. It was not a very well-made cake, but Julianne seemed oblivious to this and very pleased with herself. Dead mothers have only dead food; alive mothers have alive new fresh food. I think that cooking a meal may well be one of the early signs of recovery. The mothers in the group clearly knew this by the way they celebrated Julianne's first cake.

## SOME ISSUES INVOLVED IN WORK WITH DEPRESSED MOTHERS

Throughout this chapter, there have been the themes of a "dead" internal mother and an infant left in chaos and catastrophe. The alive, "containing," all-enveloping, at-one-with-mother state is ruptured, signaling catastrophe. In such areas of terror and pain the therapist's internal world is accessed, as a psychotic transference is awakened in the mother. Using our countertransference, the depth of feeling touches our own defenses in disorganizing and distressing ways. The work is at the level of primary maternal preoccupation and is pre-symbolic. The degree of the pain of loss awakened in the therapist is most powerful. The mother experiences her conflicts as actually relived in the therapeutic relationship with no awareness that she is repeating models of past behavior: the transference for her is "the thing in itself," the "as if" is lost. The therapist may well be experienced as charged with the emotions of an evil persecuting object. It is important to recognize that it is not only the patient, but also the therapist, who experiences the arousal of violent emotions of hate, jealousy, rivalry, and envy, as in the case of Vivienne.

Tischler (1979, 34) notes that many therapists wish to be the "good," "repairing" mother or child. This may cause us to deny the "destroying" mother, the "destroying" child, the "destroyed" mother and the "destroyed" child. Enacting a passive and neutral "analytic" stance is not useful to the depressed mother. It is too similar to the nonalive mother within. I seek to overcome this not by losing neutrality, but by being more actively alive, interpreting often and in a way that is holding. Tischler adds that the therapist's countertransference is often a shock to herself: she finds herself judgmental of the mother, seeing her as psychotic, hopeless, and in other ways not quite human. So great is the idealization of motherhood both by society and internally by ourselves. There is also the therapist's fear of the primitive energy evoked by the therapy. Sometimes, the full impact of the primitive, aggressive and sexual energies of the mother will be directed at the therapist and may stimulate our own most primitive experiences of reaching out and being accepted. There may well also be confusion in the transference as the therapist asks who am I? Am I the mother or the rejected infant?

Staying power is crucial. Attempting to do this work without adequate support is like being alone in the "madness" ourselves. It is important for anyone working in this early area of infancy to have holding, sharing, and debriefing. The group in Sydney meets for an hour and a half each week. We all work with mothers and infants. We know how hard the work is from our experience, and try to stay with the worker on a difficult case. We strive to be non-judgmental of each other's work but, even here, because of the primitive nature of the transferences and the material of this early period, we are often in conflict and carry parts of the mother's enactment, so that one will identify with the child, another with the mother's deadness, another with the therapist, and another against the therapist. I draw attention to these processes because although we are a mature group of people who have been meeting for some time, the primitive nature of the mother's material is such that it is inevitable that such enactments will be provoked. I hope these thoughts are useful to some of those working in this difficult area.

## ACKNOWLEDGMENT

"Thinking about and working with depressed mothers in the early months of their infant's life", Norma Tracey, Journal of Child Psychotherapy, volume 26, issue 2, pages 183–209. Taylor and Francis, Routledge. Copyright © Association of Child Psychotherapists, reprinted by permission of Taylor & Francis Ltd, http://www.tandfonline.com on behalf of Association of Child Psychotherapists.

## *Chapter 7*

# The Psychic Reality of Becoming a Mother

## INTRODUCTION

This chapter is about a psychic process; the process through which a woman becomes a mother. In this transition to motherhood, she mediates between a backward pull to passive being, and a forward push to active becoming; she separates from her inner idealized mother to confront the terror of death from her inner destructive one; she wins through to become an alive mother to her infant. While acknowledging the value of the father and the importance of mother father interaction, the focus here is on the internal world of woman as mother. This chapter highlights intergenerational gender processes and their effect on motherhood.

Presented in this chapter are segments of therapeutic interactions with four mothers; each portrays a mother's dramatic struggle against internal, infantile regressive forces as she pushes her way out and awakens to give birth to herself as mother. How can the therapist facilitate her working through her unresolved conflicts?

## CASE 1: WENDY

This is a weekly observation, which was part of my beginning training as a Psychoanalyst. The observation begun when the mother was in the third trimester of pregnancy with her fourth child. The observation recorded here starts ten weeks after the baby's birth. Permission to share this material has been given by the mother.

Each week, Wendy feeds her baby in my presence, but it is as if there is no baby. She connects avidly to me with her eyes, consuming me with unremitting talk. This has a desperate, voracious quality, covering any subject she thinks may interest me. I feel she gains no relief or comfort from this. Likewise, she complains her baby sucks and sucks, seems to get enough milk but appears hungry and dissatisfied even after a feed. The baby's weight gain shows an adequate milk supply. Mother and the early childhood nurse struggle for an answer. Maybe the milk is flowing too fast? She tries lying down. Maybe a dummy will help? It doesn't. The baby keeps sucking and sucking, often even vomiting up the milk afterwards because there was too much.

This observation deeply disturbs me. I am in a state of increasingly heightened tension. Is my presence intrusive, damaging her relationship with her baby? I know I am no longer an observer, but a participant in a drama of which I have no understanding. I try pushing my chair back, looking away. It makes things worse. I bring my chair close again. Unconsciously at first, then purposely, with an effort of will, I look away from her eyes, focusing my eyes on the baby at her breast. I experience her massive psychic pull as she desperately seeks my eyes again, talking even faster. I know I will not, cannot look away from the scene I have come to observe, as if my life depended on it. In determined silence, I hold my focus firmly on the feeding couple.

The mother ceases talking. The struggle ends, I relax back. She looks down at the baby at her breast. Tears come to her eyes. "I don't think I've seen this baby before." Then she says, "She's beautiful." There is silence and more tears. A little later she asks, "Did I not see Ros my older daughter either? My mother died of cancer in my last month of that pregnancy. I was so heartbroken she wasn't going to be here to see Ros, I couldn't see her either. Maybe that is why she is a remote child."

She is distressed but contained. In a gentle, sad way she speaks of a stormy adolescence with her mother, and the recovery of their relationship with Wendy's marriage, and her mother's slow death from cancer during Wendy's previous pregnancy. The sadness persists in subsequent sessions. But Wendy looks at Sarah while she feeds her now, and when she speaks, it has a resigned rather than manic quality. She has separated out from me and is focused on her baby. I experience a respect for their sacred space together. Did my presence allow her to mourn her mother, freeing her to attach to her baby?

The observation concludes twelve months later. Wendy's lack of concern at ending the observation appears to be manic denial. She is all chatter and smiles. Two months later, an urgent telephone call comes. Sarah is taking off her clothes in her sleep, and Wendy's paranoid fear is that she will choke to death on them. Her fear of Sarah's death, and the anxiety in her voice concern me. I speak at length with her, gently broaching the subject of a therapist. She telephones a few weeks later saying, "Sarah has stopped. I'm not frightened any more. Just thought I would let you know I'm OK now!" Has she resolved my leaving her? Was my presence protecting her from the internal representation of an internal destructive mother? Were the clothes imprisoning, but in trying to be free and separate, could she die? Is separation punishable by death? Wendy's husband supports and cares for her, but it is the woman's presence she needs, to find her own separateness.

## Discussion

The therapist—as a powerful, immutable holder of a space—was used by Wendy to be born as mother to her baby. She became a holder of the present to defeat the powerful pull of the past. Even as an infant, about to be born, signals the mother, Wendy as mother to her infant signaled and directed me. In that mediating space between symbiosis and separation, repetition of the past gave way. Her clinging halted, she tolerated fear, as separating from an inner idealized mother, she faced her terror or death from a persecutory one. She was alone. In that waiting space where the old was, and where the new has not yet come, is psychic pain; life and death meet. She becomes real, a real mother to her infant. There is for her then a sadness, a sadness of being. Her depressive state of acceptance is very different to postnatal depression, for in it is life and creativity. In postnatal depression is stagnation and psychic death.

## CASE 2: LEA

Dinora Pines (1982, 311) writes that in pregnancy, "primitive anxieties and conflicts arising from a woman's lifelong task of separation-individuation from her own mother may be unexpectedly revealed." There is, she adds, "a re-enactment of infantile emotional development, with libidinal aggressive and narcissistic components of the relationship to the self and to the object, altered both in the inner and outer world." The continuation of these changes in a mother in the early weeks of her baby's life is demonstrated with this next case study.

Lea is the daughter of Jewish European immigrants. She is thirty-five, a medical practitioner, living in an exclusive suburb, married to Peter, a neurologist. They have a son, age nine, and a daughter, age six, and Edward, the infant in the discussion here. Peter's obsessive demands suffocate Lea, but it is her torrid hatred of her parents and three sisters that she presents in her initial session. She felt betrayed, "robbed" of her mother's care when her sister three years younger arrived. She speaks as if this has just happened and spends her days going over and over it in her mind. In the early stages of therapy, she overwhelms the therapist with "useful" material. I wonder, are these "gifts" to appease "mother." For years of her childhood, she had given her mother gifts of being the "little mother" to her siblings, she had become her father's "son" atoning for there being no boys. But she had paid the price of the loss of her own identity, and it was some time before her sense of not being herself, of feeling cheated of her own life presented, with serious thoughts of suicide, threatening to destroy her husband, children, parents and the therapist.

A year and a half into the therapy, Lea and Peter spontaneously begin a welcomed pregnancy. Emotionally labile, Lea moves from genuine enjoyment of her fetal infant to massive anger at being a woman and tied down. Her attachment to me likewise moves from a generous sharing of the infant within—"he only dances when I am here with you"—to feeling threatened and suffocated by my presence. Sometimes she mixes up who is pregnant with whom: "I feel my existence, in the strangest way, is dependent on you. I am afraid if I kick, I will be dropped. My head know this is nonsense, but if you got run over by a bus, I would be destroyed." Other times she claims no need of me at all.

We agree that she take her own time to return after the birth. She telephones twice from the hospital. I am aware her focus is on her own fragile and dazed state, not her baby. She speaks of turbulence with calm oily water in spaces between. She gives me a lengthy, intensely detailed description of the birth, but again with little mention of her baby. She chooses to return to therapy the day after arriving home. This is very unusual. In her first session Lea repeats her story of the birth. It is a long and painful birth, halted for hours in the final stage of dilation. Despite all her effort, she could not give birth. She gives in, asking for an epidural, and then a caesarean. A remarkable midwife comes on the scene, "Look dear, there is no reason you can't do this. Let me talk you through it." They work hard. Edward is born.

Relating every detail of the birth is a normal post-birth phenomenon, but when Lea tells it to me for the fifth time, I say, "Lea, what are you trying to tell me? What am I not grasping?" "I don't know," she says. "I feel as if I'm missing something." Next morning in the shower a psychic push comes . "Norma, you lovely bitch!" she cries through clenched teeth, pushing and pushing as she emotionally makes her psychic way through. "Norma, I loved and hated you so much in that extraordinary time." Do life and death, love and hate meet at birth? I ask myself. Does the depressive position begin at birth? Is the meeting of life and death at birth the beginning of the depressive position for both mother and baby?

Some weeks later, Lea asks a strange question: "Norma. Why are sick people happier than normal ones, why are sane people sad? My husband becomes interested in me only when I fail, then he can take over. My mother would be thrilled on the other hand if my marriage failed, because then she could take over. I feel as if I want to fail." After this conversation, Lea arrives at each session increasingly beside herself. She says her baby is failing to thrive. She does not have enough milk for him. She feels l have failed her since she is begging for answers, and I sit in determined silence. She breaks down, saying she feels insecure and unsure of herself and terribly frightened. All the work we have done together has been a waste of time. At first, I am concerned, again wondering, "What am I missing?" I could see nothing. Gradually, her rage toward the mother/me, becomes clear. She races to the early childhood sister, panics her into canceling all of her other home visits to spend a full afternoon with Lea. The local doctor spends hours with her, eventually referring her to the pediatrician. He is at first calm, but succumbs to her panic, saying if the baby does not gain weight within five days, she must wean immediately. In her sessions with me, she pulls and pushes at me to deliver answers. "Weren't you the specialist in this area?" she mocks, knowing from her pediatrician that I have a reputation in this area. I sit firm and mostly silent. She glares at me, saying if she sits and waits for me, her baby will die of starvation. The healthcare sister, feeling desperate, says, "I wonder if you shouldn't see a counselor dear?" I tell Lea she has one, and ask why is she doing this? Lea becomes more stubbornly desperate, filling the baby now with solids. I worry, "Am I starving her, what is going on?" Is she perhaps desperate to fail in order to show me up as a failure? I find the answer in her as the little girl, replaced by a baby sister, and forced to grow up overnight. Can she have so confused the past and present that she is in fact in rivalry with her own baby? Has she mixed up the baby with herself, and is now desperate that the mother take it over? The unconscious is unknowing of time and persons; it has no discrimination.

I interpret: "You run to me, you run to the health visitor, you run to the general practitioner, the pediatrician, your husband. You know what, I ask—where is the mother in you? I think those answers you scream for from us, you have inside you. You are the mother." She cries out that she is cracking up, that she is desperate, that I am cruel and unsympathetic. She storms out. She will not be "returning," she says as she leaves.

That night, Lea hears her baby cry. She turns over to go to sleep, ignoring the cry. Someone inside her awakens in fright. She realizes she has been turning over and not responding to him each night. "It was a terrible moment. I realized it was me, all me. Oh God! I've been leaving him hungry." She gets up. She feeds him. For the next three days she feeds him whenever he cries. There is only him and her now. She drops all visits to health professionals, but continues her sessions. Sadly sober, she says, "I didn't want to get up and feed him. I was starving my own baby." Edward thrives well from this point on. Lea continued in therapy for some years.

## Discussion

With Lea, I am aware of the quality of the regressive pull and its power. In defeating this, she takes back her own projections, owning her part in the living narrative. In doing so she owns her infant, awakening to herself as a mother. There is a depression following this insight, but it is a healthy depression, more of a depressive position that is creative.

What is the special nature of the therapeutic interaction that allows such changes? The elucidation of this begins with long-held ideas of dynamic and dialectic. Ogden (1985, 133) gives a precise definition of a dialectic "as a process in which two opposing concepts each create, inform, preserve and negate the other, each standing in a dynamic (ever changing) relationship with the other." The dialectical process moves towards integration, but integration is never complete; each integration creates a new dialectical opposition and a new dynamic tension. The therapeutic action frees the movement between opposites. This movement between opposites is present in every stage of living.

Maizels (1985, 188) writes of "a psychological tendency in many ways corresponding to Freud's conception of the death instinct, [that pulls] towards achieving a permanent state of non-tension, non-effort, sleep, peace, passivity and oblivion." He writes of an opposite tendency "characterized by desires for autonomy, independence and the overcoming of frustrations in the external world through effort. These two tendencies are often felt to be in a state of conflict, particularly prior to the working through of the depressive position" (Maizels 1985, 188). The anxiety relating to this conflict, "can only be corrected by the availability, and eventually internalization of a mediating object" (Maizels 1985, 189).

Feder (1980, 164) says, "These opposites exist before conception when the mutually attracted heterosexual couple awaken and stimulate in each other a series of interpersonal, ambivalent and contradictory conflicts, usually unconscious, but as expression always of their intra-psychic dilemmas towards pregnancy. . . . There is evidence of 'procreative joy' as opposed to 'procreative panic.'" For every woman, pregnancy, birth and each stage of her life with her partner and infant offers a reawakening of that stage of her own existence. With this comes another chance at resolution.

There is for each woman rivalry with her mother, and a healthy wish to be like her; anger at being woman and maternal, and gratitude for this gift of motherhood; fear of an internal mother taking her baby for revengeful reprisal, and an image of a protective mother, who secures her in her role. It is the mediation of these dialectics that allows a woman to become mother.

There is in any psychic growth a breaking with the status quo, an old set or structure, to make space for a new one. Pick (1985) writes of seduction by the patient's internal material to repeat old patterns. When this occurs, it strengthens the status quo, and blocks change. This backward pull of forceful, impulse-ridden demands lacks reflection. There is a demand for immediacy of satisfaction, a desperation, a push from within, rather than the sense of being goal oriented. Relief is sought for the sake of relief. It lacks any other purpose. There is a desire to escape responsibility and demand another's action, rather than taking action on one's own. Self is absent.

The therapist's refusal to meet these demands helps her surrender them and face her ownership of her own actions. The change that comes with pregnancy is well documented by Dinora Pines (1982). These changes reach a series of crises in the first weeks of motherhood. Letting go of old identifications, and old ways of acting, is fearsome. In the chaos is the terror of loss, facing of the fear of death, waiting for her own psychic birth as a mother.

The moment itself needed grasping. Lea gathered the confusion and anxiety of a nursing sister, a general practitioner, a pediatrician and her husband to avoid owning her own truth, murderously furious at having to take care of her own baby as when her mother had a new baby of her own. Her hatred toward her mother/me was a hatred of herself as an adult woman and mother. The rage caused by the frustration of the therapist's refusal to have her answers, made her turn in to seek and own her own answers. Hate met love; her mediator awakened; she could find her own answers. There was a new center of power, albeit initially fragile in a changed inner-world structure. This center of power is motherhood.

Interpretations are the result of processing and reflecting, not only on the patient's emotions but one's own. Thus, they are born from the depth of the therapist's and the patient's deepest unconscious interactions. Change occurs not only for the patient but for the therapist at the deepest level. Two people psychically move; two people grow. While the therapist knows about bearing the unbearable, and thinking the unthinkable, the creative movement is the intercourse between the two. No amount of training can cause or predict this or make it any easier. It is a new step for the therapist and patient every time.

Grinberg (1990) gives meaning to a special kind of response that he called "projective counteridentification." He describes a passive receptivity in the therapist that allows a situation in which she ceases to be herself, turning unavoidably into what the patient wants her to be. I suggest that in the action of psychic change the therapist takes an active stand, breaking this passive acceptance of a patient-nominated role. Breaking with projective identification, means refusing the given role in the internal drama, and creating a new role of one's own. In psychic change, the therapist disillusions the patient's omnipotence by not accepting the projection. The drama is no longer enacted. It returns to its own loner world where it can be contained and processed.

When Lea stopped projecting her anxiety and terror, a special action to do with ownership of her projections seemed to take place. Lea accepted herself as the center of her being, rather than demanding the therapist be that center. She mediated her own comments, owned her own projections, acknowledged the limitations of her human condition; above all, she owned her baby. She faced loss, was separate, and became her own person.

In summary, the processes of psychic change as described here are an exposure of a dialectic; an immutable holding of a neutral stance to free a dynamic between opposites. This neutral stance resists infantile regressive demands; accepting one's own emotions of rage, allowing love and hate to meet and a new psychic presence to be born.

## CASE 3: LAURA

Laura married late in life. She is a book editor, and is respected for her quiet, unobtrusive attention to detail. She married James in her mid-thirties. She had a severe depressive breakdown five years before she came to see me and had not worked since. She sees herself as recovered, plans this baby, welcoming and enjoying her pregnancy and the birth as an expression of her recovery. A sensitive and vulnerable woman, she thinks deeply at times; at other times she becomes phased out and autistic-like. James is a music teacher and a Zen follower who, with his wife, believes in simplicity of living and abhors the trappings of modern life. They have a harpsichord; they do not have a television. James and Laura are like twin souls, devoted to each other.

On arriving for her first session, Laura is beside herself. With no known diagnosis, her ten-day-old baby has not sucked since birth. Feeding him minute expressed amounts with a bottle takes over an hour, then the rest of the feed is through a permanently inserted nasal tube. Laura's trauma begins with her discharge from hospital without her baby—"like my arm pulled out of its socket and left behind." On another occasion, she describes this separation as feeling "disemboweled as if I had lost my own middle." She sees herself as a failure for not demanding that she stay with her baby. She sees this failure as a crime, his illness as a death sentence. She looks autistic-like, strained, with periods of intense emotion interspersed with periods of blankness. These have no links, and are apparently disconnected. James arrives for the session later. He is very supportive, yet angry and hurt. "Living has always been a struggle," he says. "Being alive is a costly business. I always feared the bad guys would win over the good guys. Now they have. I don't have hope in anything or anyone."

These early sessions with Laura are hard. I spend every moment validating her feelings, since everyone is saying she is mad. I think it is normal to be mad with a baby like this. A "truthful" pediatrician terrifies her. He tells her the baby may never suck, but he has no diagnosis. Mostly I just sit with her, this dazed, silent, disorientated woman. Sometimes I very gently touch her pain, and then a storm of horrendous crying racks her body, stopping as suddenly as it began. Laura returns to her phased-out, dazed appearance. I feel as if Timothy is dead even though alive during those first few months, and so is his mother. She is always present with him, but to my horror, they both look moribund when I see them together.

Laura is in terror of her own monsters; they claim her baby for death, not for life. They tell her: "You only deserve a damaged baby; this is your punishment for daring to attempt to be happy and have a baby." Laura grew up believing she has no rights to a husband, marriage, or a baby of her own. The sensitive James and his love have entered her life like a miracle. Now all of it has gone bad. In the beginning, she clings to me in an idealizing state. I tolerate this, knowing she needs it, to defeat a destructive mother within.

Eventually, initial thoughts of punishment give way to a healthier protest. "It's unfair, it's unfair, it's unfair! Why has everybody else in the world got a healthy baby except me? I can't be that bad!" She is angry enough at one stage for me to ask her if she is in danger of hurting herself or her baby. "No! I would never hurt my baby, never touch a hair of his head, but I am angry with him for showing me up as such a bad person and such a failure."

The tests went on, revealing nothing. The pediatrician is angry. He cannot find answers. Laura and James justifiably feel blamed. A transfer is made to a large children's hospital. Laura lives in. James visits nightly. The diagnosis is bulbar palsy. He needs an operation to put a feeding tube bypassing his mouth straight through as a permanent fixture into his stomach. They see me daily. They are devastated.

At discharge, Laura has lost all confidence. The ward worries about her competence and the pediatrician telephones me at home at night seeking assurance that it is safe to discharge her. A battle ensues between her and the ward about whose baby this is. She wants her baby discharged. They want her to return every twenty-four hours to see how she is managing. Laura's anxiety and constant expression of fear has entered them. They become possessive and protective of the baby. The ward social worker comes to the rescue. Timothy goes home.

Laura and James take Timothy to a holiday beach about 100 kilometers away. She tells me of her dream of walking with her baby on the seashore, knowing she, James and Timothy are at last secure together. Timothy has other ideas. Timothy screams and screams for the first time in his life. He angrily pushes the bottle away. They try to use the tube, but his screams cause stomach contractions, and the milk shoots out of the tube. They go to the local hospital and see the early childhood sister. Nothing is physically wrong. They telephone me during this ordeal. Laura tells me she has given up in despair. She will never be able to look after her baby; she will bring him back to the children's hospital. "They were right. I can't do it," she says in bitter resignation.

James imagines carrying his baby in his arms and, with Laura, walking into the sea and disappearing. I say, "Timothy's screaming is surely better than his lying there half-dead as he was before. Now that he is with his mother and father he can protest and express rage for all the intrusions he has suffered. Hold him and hold him and let him know you can survive it. This is something no hospital can do, only the two of you." Laura telephones later, "We are holding him, we are in the middle of his nightmare with him." Then the screaming seems to be abating. There is another call. "He has stopped crying and drunk the whole bottle. We think this is because he has got his anger out. James and I think it is a miracle." The tube is never used again. It is removed some months later.

For Laura and James this event is baptism by fire. It creates an extraordinary bond with Timothy. He does well. James begins therapy and Laura continues with her therapy once a week.

## Discussion

When a newborn baby is ill, terrible feelings of self-blame, guilt, impotence, and of being cursed leave a mother feeling persecuted and depleted. A negative, destructive, internal mother appears to triumph over a good, life-giving one. There is a feeling of punishment and revenge for her desire to become a mother. In the space where the pain is more than she can bear, she breaks down, defending with a shell that in fact protects a now unfeeling, non-living space. The devastation for a mother, when she fails to be what Bollas (1987) called a transformational object for her infant is terrible. The new mother needs to experience herself as a transformational object. When she cannot, a mother's sense of impotence and failure destroys her internal image of herself as potent and capable of warding off illness, evil, and destruction. The privacy, stillness, and special culture born out of an interaction between mother and infant is impinged on. It becomes the stillness of death, not of waiting. The premature separation is "an arm wrenched from its socket." For her husband, the father, the fracturing of his illusion of creating a protective shield is no less devastating.

The dynamic between a dreamt-of baby, a dreaded baby, and a real baby is disturbed when the reality of a "damaged" one exists. Normally at birth, there is both disappointment and celebration. For here is the baby as it is, not as it appeared in the dream, not as dreaded in the nightmare. The reality of a thriving infant gives hope of a future. It is this hope that sustains a mother as she mourns the loss of the infant from her womb. A mother whose baby is ill does not feel "full of grace" or "blessed amongst women" or "blessed in the fruit of her womb." She reels as Laura did, empty, cursed in the "fruit of her womb," and a failure "amongst women." Her dream of a future for her baby is lost. Instead, she has a despair of death or permanent damage. How does this affect her journey through what Winnicott (1984b) has called "primary maternal preoccupation"? Primary maternal preoccupation protects against primary maternal persecution, a term coined by Raphael-Leff. (1991). Winnicott's understanding of primary maternal preoccupation may well be a protection from the persecution of the mother's own murderous feelings towards her baby as separate. She wants him fused and back in her womb. Her preoccupation protects her baby from the persecution of his own internal turmoil, which is too chaotic for his vulnerable state to hold. Her preoccupation protects him from the persecution or extremes of his own bodily states, such as hunger and discomfort. Her preoccupation protects him from the persecution from the outside world, such as intrusion from temperature extremes, noise, and any danger. All this was lost for Laura. She could not protect her baby or herself from internal or external persecutors. In her husband's words, "the baddies were winning." Winnicott (1984b) writes of mothers who enter preoccupation but find great difficulty in moving out. A mother moves out when her baby is thriving, and she feels released by him. Her baby's crying, traumatic though it was, brought them to life as a family. The living-out of the trauma, caused by this little infant's howling response, heralded a possibility of living, although it felt like dying. Catastrophic crisis and psychic birth are extremely close.

For Laura and James, it was a test of whether they could hold on when the concept of themselves as caring capable parents was so damaged. There was a question of will the crying end? Neither parents nor infants in the earliest preoccupation states have memory. The powerful immediacy of emotions means that each event is in itself the whole. This is so for infant and mother. If he is crying, they only know a crying infant. They lose the mental concept of a baby that does not cry. The existential nature of this requires hedonistic immediacy of response. This makes the anxiety of the moment enormous. Immediacy of feeding predicts the whole future. When a baby is fine and well fed, a mother will be elated with hope of the future. If he rejects a single feed, it may be enough to foresee a disastrous future, and despair may take over.

In actively caring for her baby a mother takes control of the future, thus directing fate, not being its victim. She experiences her potency. She sustains the experience as well as the illusion of transforming her baby's world, eventually surrendering this to settle for being good enough. Laura found her strength as a holding mother so that her infant had an object where his emotions of protest and rage could be placed. His crying asked them all to hear him and may well have been his breakout from trauma.

There is a special autonomous space where the mother and baby reside. The father is the protector of this space. There is a line to do with mother-infant autonomy, which the therapist can never cross. A therapist can try to avoid this by keeping her neutral interpretive stance, focusing on the mother and the mother's internal baby, thus never competing for care of the external one. However, when another enters the circle of the mother and infant, their space is violated, and there is competition with her for the baby. A mother may well experience any intrusion, as Laura did, as a rivaling caretaker, as a robbing mother. Laura had to awaken as mother to battle for her role. Her space with her baby had not totally recovered. She has only let me see him twice, once in hospital, and then when he was eighteen months old. She found her mother-in-law's handling of him intrusive. There was justification here, but the amniotic sac in her mind remained vulnerable for a long time. A mother may be able to identify with a good ward team and experience them as part of her. But this needs active, direct involvement, and staff need the capacity to deal with persecuted and persecutory feelings. There is a frightening message for an intensive care ward here: they may save an infant's life but, without respect for the mother's autonomy, they may leave her psychically childless. When Laura lost her autonomy with her infant, she lost her protection from her own persecutory internal mother. When I gave her my holding and containing, Laura could introject this, making her intolerable journey tolerable. My containing space for her anger, her rage, and her turbulent emotions helped her create a holding space for Timothy to express his. The structure of a therapy, its frame, the therapist simply being present, and her capacity to listen and to hear, was a shock absorber for the mother's trauma. It gave her a psychic skin and, in it, a space where she could go mad and recover.

## CASE 4: SUZIE

For the mother, pregnancy and birth is a transitional period, and can result in what Dinora Pines (1990) calls a "crisis of maturation." As is the case in any transitional period in human life, "uneasy conflicts belonging to past developmental stages are revived, thus, the old ambivalent identifications may be resolved, and new and more peaceful relationships take place" (Pines 1990, 301). Pregnancy and birth are real as well as psychic events, presenting a unique opportunity for past traumas to be exposed and healed. A woman is motivated to "get it right" for her and her baby. With Suzie, in her pregnancy birth crisis, there was a chance to open old wounds and to repair and reconstruct. Suzie's pregnancy gave the therapist a chance to be "pregnant" with her, a chance for her to come to life from a psychic death caused by her mother's death.

At our first meeting, Suzie is two months pregnant. She is in her mid-thirties and has abandoned her already deteriorating two-year relationship, refusing to abort. Suzie's mother died of cancer when she was twelve, her father when she was eighteen years old. She gave the impression of being poor and not very intelligent. Both these impressions are wrong. Her parent's left her a multimillionaire, her dullness is a mask, as is her gross obesity. I offer Suzie therapy four times a week, with an initial trial period. She accepts, refusing the couch, and limiting the therapy to the time of her pregnancy.

The countertransference and response to Suzie are powerful. To my amazement, the end of each session provokes a fear of termination, like a fetus clinging to life. Both psychically and emotionally she gives a fetal image, a fat blob, sitting there with a narcissistic control over everything. My fear is clearly hers, but it would be fatally premature to interpret. Suzie's family spoiled her as an infant and small child. In return, she did not cry, protest, or move. She is the same now. Her mother imagined a full-term phantom pregnancy before her conception with Suzie, yet she was often away after her birth. When she died, Suzie was filled with valium each day, not to relieve her distress, but to make sure she never had any. This changed to a glass of brandy, poured and waiting each afternoon after school. She remembers being drunk daily. There was a series of maids. Her father, often drunk, lost awareness of her. Much later, she reveals these as years of starvation, aloneness, and destitution. The addictive defenses against psychic pain began then and continue today in the form of compulsive bingeing and constant buying.

Everything she brings to the therapy has the same theme of being taken over and being powerless to stop it. She said even if she begins a sentence, it is terminated by the intrusion of another person, their ideas being substituted for hers. A recurring nightmare, begun at the age of four, reveals a narrative of self-appropriation at an early age. In the dream, she is to take care of a baby sister with an enlarged head. She takes her to a circus. There the baby is mistaken for a cake, cut up, and sold for eating. Suzie's horrified screams of protest are ignored. She is powerless. She awakens in fright.

I have strong reactive feelings when with her. I also feel powerless often losing the sense of who I am—mother, baby, either, both? Later I am well in touch with a murderous mother, who can terminate me. Suzie is grateful I survive. I know I must, even when the sessions are totally deadening. I begin to dread the deadening in me in each session. "Excuse me, I think you're going to sleep again," she says, unemotionally. She becomes stronger about it and her messages begin to awaken me. I ask, "Is she bringing her mother back to life?" She says, "I think so, but if I stand up for myself, I think something terrible is going to happen to me or my family." As I fight the deadness of the sessions, she fights a deadness inside her. One day, I realize for the first time that the fear of termination is gone. In the same session Suzie says, "I know

I am connected to you now, and I know I will be continuing therapy." Then unaware of any link, since she has no awareness of links, she says, "This morning when they did the scan, I heard the baby's heartbeat for the first time." However, for Suzie, beginning to live is terrifying. Nightmares come. She lies in terror, paralyzed, as black spiders climb on her. There is no voice with which to cry, and I actually feel as if I am pregnant with her. The most minute hint of sadness passes between us. Then I begin to feel as if I am suffocating again. I begin to yawn in her sessions. "You're yawning," she tells me, without emotion. In later sessions the yawning stops. As is the pattern of our work, each sign of life reverts back to deadness. This nothing-deadness fills our sessions. She breaks the silence saying, "This nothing is how I have lived most of my life." She tells me of being aware of her skin being so thick (fat thick) that she fears they/we cannot cut through to the baby. My interpretations are experienced as a sharp refined blade cutting through false self. Then an itching begins. It is one month until the birth of her baby. This itching pursues and persecutes her morning, noon and night. One day, Suzie is livid with rage toward me for the first time. She shakes from head to foot. I have convinced her, she says, that this itching is psychological. This morning her specialist said her liver assays showed elevated results. The baby could die. The itching is because of this. I had strongly stressed that she should have the itching checked medically. Far from experiencing anger at her accusation, I am elated. She is angry, alive, and terrified of death. I am now part of a powerful paranoid process. Suzie is in a state of anguished terror. At a cousin's wedding one night, she faces her raging sense of aloneness. She feels massive envy towards everyone there with a partner. She stays up all night with the itching, experiencing it change into rage and hate. The following morning the itch stops and never returns. The results from her liver assays remained above normal, but later fell.

Suzie chooses to come to therapy right up to the day of birth. We have an agreement that she will decide after the birth if she wants to return. It is important to her that this subject remains taboo, her choice entirely. I am warned that one mention of it will ensure she does not return. She telephones four days after the birth. It was a terrible birth. She shook as if convulsed for two hours, developed a bacterial infection, and the baby is still in the intensive care nursery. Her voice is monotonal and uninviting.

Two days later, she telephones again. She is happy. Her baby is in her arms feeding. She is going home. I will hear from her again. I feel lost during this time, hovering in doubt. Will I see her again? What a strange way to go. I wait. Three weeks later, she says can she visit, just once. She decides she will come once a week. Seeing me becomes very distressing for her. She is all right when away from me, but for two days before the session and two days after she is in great distress. In unbearable pain of aloneness, she hugs her baby, dances to her music with him, and binges. She knows this is to do with the pain inside her. I present to my colleagues in our weekly case group discussion. I am paranoid. I feel they do not help or understand me. I experience the remarks of this group, for which I have respect and attachment, as judgmental and unsympathetic. They see me as inadequate: "You are dead for her; she has not found you since the birth." I am in psychic agony. I speak with each in turn the following day. Something sorts itself out in my mind to do with my autonomy, with my patient, and giving me space. They agree. In hindsight, I think we have enacted the transference between her and myself. I have given them my despair. I think if her living means her mother must die, then there is no space for her to live. Once I grasp this, we enter Suzie's psychotic grief, an encapsulated area of intense psychic pain. The movement into and out of this grief is of long duration. I provide a non-intruding presence where pain can be held. I know her pain. I can freely talk about it with her. But the pain I feel I know is mine. She is now feeling her own pain. A rich phantasy overtakes me in a session. Her twelve-year-old self is running down empty corridors looking for an absent mother, howling as she faces that there is no mother there for her. I tell her about the image in my mind. The room fills with howls, primitive howls of agonizing loss. The howling fills the session. She sits in an unbearable pain. We bear it. There is no cover-up now. "My mother's death," she says. "I have been dead ever since, haven't I?" Suzie becomes seriously paranoid. She sits up all night fearing cot death. This is an exaggerated primary maternal preoccupation. It continues for some days. We weather it together. Then she has a dream. In the dream, she is happily bathing her baby, his head resting on her wrist. She falls asleep and awakens with a start, to find he is blue. In the dream there is a frantic effort to resuscitate him and much anger with herself for falling asleep. I interpret her as having awakened to take care of her baby.

In another dream, she is visiting a doctor friend and they look down at her baby. To her horror, there is a deep scar right down his right cheek. She screams out to the doctor: "What is this?" The doctor's ominous reply is, "This is the depression he has inherited from you."

Suzie's depression then gives way to a mighty rage at the years of her life she feels she has not lived—the years of which she feels robbed. She demands she finish her own sentences and think her own thoughts, to the consternation of her family and friends who are trying to adjust to a different Suzie. She begins to own herself as an angry, but alive, infant. As she does, she is no longer "innocent" to anger and attack from others. Her baby thrives. Therapy continues.

## Discussion

García Badaracco (1992, 218) writes, "There is an interrelationship and simultaneity between psychic change, anxiety and insight. Change and insight are two phases of a dialectical process. A change allows an insight, and the insight may give further rise to change. For significant psychic changes to occur, there must be processes of identificatory restructuring, which are necessarily accompanied by psychotic anxieties, and this explains why they are so powerfully resisted."

I think Suzie never had a space in which to live. Emotional and intellectual appropriation was obvious from infancy. Even physical movement seemed unacceptable. Once, during a session, I smiled back at her baby as it looked over. Suzie burst into tears: "This is my session; I have little enough time with you as it is." This was a rivalrous Suzie child. At a more mature level, she was the guardian of her space with her baby. "You promised you would not interfere with whatever I do with my baby. I know I can trust you not to do this." I did not look at her external baby after this, except at her express invitation. She was to be mother, the active one. The risk of appropriation seemed potently present.

Bion (1977) makes sense of how the mother's absence, not her presence, creates an experience or a phantasy of an internal persecuting mother. Absence intrudes more than presence because in the emptiness and hunger is a living pain that brings up the image of a bad persecutory mother. The absent mother is both a bad mother and an over-idealized mother. There is no real mother to allow separation and mediation. Did Suzie also "die" to satisfy her? Or did she "die" because the pain was unbearable with no one to share it? Although my caring presence offered some safety, a negative robbing mother becomes a real-life enactment of dramatically terrifying proportions. Suzie stayed up all night with her baby, trying to protect him against her own absent dead destructive mother.

For Suzie, being alive is much worse than being dead. She must recognize the robber, the murderer, as a part of her denied, introjected, retaliatory mother. She must overcome the dead mother, pulling her towards passive death, and take hold of this alive mother here, who psychically defeats death and offers life. She must, most of all, suffer the pain of being truly alone. The reactivation of previous psychotic experiences to do with her mother's death, again seemed to require of me a strong, firmly holding, unafraid self. Then together we could tolerate the intolerable. I could hold her terror. She could then have her own life and her own insight.

My previous work to do with trauma (Tracey 1991) relates well to Suzie. In it is postulated that when a negative pain from an absence intrudes and becomes greater than the positive hallucination, then, instead of neutralization, there is archaic denial and repression. There is no thought, no storing of a model, no abstraction, and an empty space is available for any occupancy from without. There is, therefore, a passive failure to see or understand danger. The space where one waits for the person to be themselves is a devastated no life area. One must battle with this no-life space, as Suzie and I as her therapist did, to reach life. This means she must suffer her insufferable psychic pain. It means processing the pain to small tolerable doses, instead of being flooded by the pain.

In normal development, psychic pain occurs when new cohesion, a new coming together in order to become a realization, demands the surrender of the old. The waiting, the agreeing to wait, and the capacity to wait mean facing loss and turbulence and experiencing the emptiness. This we were to repeat over and over with Suzie. It is more painful to live and face loss, than to be psychically dead.

The therapist in this internal drama of psychic change provides an immutable holding space. Here the mother can surrender old infantile regressive needs, to become. This becoming takes place through a deep interactive process, a relationship reaching its peak with the heat of the here and now. Acting out is interpreted; rage, envy and destructiveness are tolerated; the terror of death in surrendering old identifications is acknowledged; hate and anger from frustration are allowed; projections are re-owned; psychic pain is suffered; insight is experienced; the sadness of being is accepted; a woman is born as mother to her infant.

# *Chapter 8*

# The Autistic Core in Aboriginal Trauma

The catastrophe that befell the Australian Aboriginal peoples through colonialism is reflected through stolen children, disbanded communities, and appropriated land . This trauma resulted in their dislocation from culture and loss of generational continuity. It is a tragedy that leaves many Aboriginals devoid of protection from within their own psyche and the current world in which they live. When they were cut off from their culture, community and earth place, meaning became lost for them. Far more seriously, what they also lost was their ancient ritualistic or customary ways of dealing with trauma. They were no longer in touch with their own significant meaningful culture and myths.

The Dreaming and Dadirri are two significant gifts from ancient Aboriginal peoples that provide valuable insights for treating trauma. In the ancient concept of the Dreaming, Aboriginal people imbued the external world, and events in it, with emotional meaning born from internal world symbols and narratives. Ancient Aboriginal culture healed trauma through Dadirri, known by modern Aboriginal people as the "healing circle." Dadirri is a ritualized form of "deep listening," not an ordinary witnessing but an empathic psychic action. It is what we now call psychotherapy. To understand the important contribution Dadirri can make to treating trauma, we first need to explore what breakdowns occur in trauma.

## BREAKDOWN IN TRAUMA

It is important to understand the difference between "breakdown" and "break-out." As I wrote in Chapter 1, in extreme cases, such as trauma in early infancy or childhood, or severe adult trauma, if the defense becomes concretized, a psychotic "pocket" or core or dead internal mind-state may result. The "autistic cut-out" is a normal primitive defense, working to protect the person from overstimulation. But this means emotion is unable to be experienced, pain is unable to be suffered, meaning is lost, and the "thingifying" or concretization causes loss of internal reverie and empathy. If this autistic defense does not hold, the "breakdown" is worse. Chaos, envy and rage overflow, with ensuing primitive enactment, which may include criminality. Aboriginal people now have the problem of serious addiction, which may initially be an effort to quell the nightmare of such mad emotions, enacted as violence, rape, murder and suicide. In such cases, they have no internal holding boundaries to protect themselves or others from the primitive overflow.

"Trauma breakout" is quite different. It allows the movement out of this psychotic autistic defense, sometimes expressed as a scream of existence; one dares to experience and suffer the suffering, in the suffering. This is a recovery from trauma, an explosion of primitive emotions that could not be accessed because of the strength of the autistic defense (Tracey 2000). It is the holding of this "breakout," very different from the term "breakdown," that allows for the restoration of health. After this initial "flood" of trauma breakout, the dosage and the timing of responses are extremely relevant and require an empathic awareness on the part of the therapist.

In ancient Aboriginal tribes in Australia, this process took place between a person and a group and is called Dadirri. The group's presence allowed the pain to be expressed, empathized with, and suffered in a way that processed it. This is Dadirri. Recovery in the therapeutic process is similar. Psychoanalytic therapy requires a space where suffering of the suffering in the suffering can occur. It also requires careful monitoring and negotiation—in terms of timing and dosage—of the ego's ability to tolerate, use and process that suffering. The quality of the group's presence in Dadirri is similar to what a mother does for her infant in reverie.

The "new" form of therapy used in psychoanalytic thought and work is modeled on the older form of the Dadirri that was lost to the Aboriginal people when they lost their own culture. An Aboriginal health worker in my team described it best: "I thought this psychoanalytic stuff was a lot of shit. Now I listen to it carefully and it fits so perfectly for our people. It is in the same place as our Dreaming."

In her book *Trauma Trails, Recreating Song Lines* (2002), Judy Atkinson sensitively deals with trauma caused by abuse, alcoholism, and drug dependency. Sharing their stories, contributors demonstrate the Aboriginal gift to the nation—Dadirri—listening to one another, and showing the way it provides a way forward. By inviting non-Indigenous people to sit with them in the circle, sharing stories, listening to and learning from each other, song lines emerge of a courageous journey, pointing us in the direction of change and healing.

From this capacity to dream evolves meaning. This meaning, expressed through mythology and symbols, becomes a wisdom transmitted and transposed through generations by Aboriginal elders in oral and cave art forms. An ancient spirituality gives historic continuity to the inner self; it links to ancestors and elders in the past; it provides a sense of belonging in the present living community. It creates a link from the internal world to the external world, giving meaning to the relationship between the person and nature, and the inner person and the environment. It gives value to selfhood, community, and culture. The rules or laws that bind these meanings become sacred, and the symbols born from them are precious, creating a boundary within which to contain and hold meaning. From here, all sense of internal and external chaos and disharmony can be tolerated, until a self in harmony within and without is experienced.

Does dislocation from this Dreaming, this spiritual, cultural base, affect the way a people experience themselves? The trauma of dislocation for Aboriginals as a people kills meaning, nullifies the internal illusion, destroys the capacity to sublimate into art and story, and destroys the psychic binding that symbol formation gives. It denudes the experience of a living self; the person experiences themselves as a "no person," in an autistic defense that protects against overwhelming internal chaos. Dreams become real; they concretize. The Dreaming is lost and replaced by a nightmare. We think here of a dead mother and, therefore, a dead fetal self. This is psychosis.

## IN THE BEGINNING: BEFORE THE DREAMING, PRECREATIVE SPACE

At the core of the personality is a particular psychic space, a precreative, primordial abyss. It is the nothingness, the nowhere space, appearing in most religions as the primary abyss: as the King James Bible has it, "and the earth was without form, and void" (Genesis 1:2). This space was there before all creative experiencing, before all ambivalence; in the Tao,"it is before is and is not" (Mitchell 1992, 21). In Hebrew it is known as "tehom"—the abyss or "bottomless sea." It is not a static space, for there is a dialectical movement to and from it in every living experience. Old patterns of being are surrendered to allow return to the abyss, yet paradoxically for the first time, and from there emerges the potential to be born psychically anew. This dynamic is a continuum from birth to death, from womb to tomb (Tracey 2009, 1025). Rose Ungunmerr, an Aboriginal elder, in the introduction to *Dadirri: The Spring Within*, writes, "It is the place before we were born, before we were in our mother's womb" (quoted in Farrelly 2003, viii). When trauma occurs, there is another psychic space—the dark abyss resulting from unresolved trauma. It has no growth, no movement; in that space death becomes more active than life, annihilating of life. At the center is terror. The mind also closes down in a physical sense; in trauma, the amygdala closes down from the hippocampus. This creates the autistic-like space, the nothing space where nothing grows. Aboriginal people appeared to have an understanding of the concept of this dead "no-faith" space. In the Kimberley region of Western Australia, paintings by the Wandjina tribe of Aboriginal people are re-enlivened by present-day artists reworking them. This is the view of an elder quoted in *Australian Dreaming* (2005):

> I don't know all what happened to you, but all your spirit has gone out of you. No men or women watch over you, for the people who belong to this place—my aunties, sisters, fathers and grannies—they are all dead now. Only I, who belong to another place came to visit you, but you are lonely for all those people who died, and your spirit has gone away now. Because you are looking all dull—you are not looking bright—I'll try and draw you. I will try and put new paint on you people. Don't get wild! Don't send rain! You must be very glad because I will make your eyes like new. My eye it has life, and your eye has life too, because I make it new. (quoted in Isaacs 2005, 71)

## THE DREAMING

In the Red Centre of Australia, the mythic landscape has existed for countless millennia. As Cowan (1994, 22) writes, the Aboriginal people "have sought to reconcile themselves to an outwardly barren environment by living a rich imaginal life inspired by the power of the myth."

Cowan adds that the Dreaming network of tribal boundaries, languages, sacred songs, rituals, and ceremonies held Aboriginal culture together. He tells that in the northern region of Australia, a sacred cult known as Kunapipi still preserves the mythogenic reality of the Sacred Mother, the perpetually pregnant woman. On the one hand, she is regarded as a fertility figure; on the other hand, she is linked to the Rainbow Serpent as a symbol of abundance and renewal. To talk of her is to engage in a dialogue with all the mothers of the world. Her form may be that of the many-breasted Diana of Ephesus, a plump effigy vessel from Minoan Crete, or the Egyptian goddess Nut, overreaching the sky. She may be Kali, Rati, or Venus. Whatever her image, Kunapipi embodies a principle of fecundity that transcends all her many manifestations. She is both female in her creative, nurturing phase, and male in her seminal, ordering phase. Combining mysteriously with the Rainbow Serpent, we see vulva and phallus merge into one generative organ in her being: "She is Sophia, the 'spirit and the bride' of the Apocalypse, the process by which all things are spiritualized by the 'living waters' that she represents" (Cowan 1994, 22).

The elder, Rose Ungunmerr (she is now known as Miriam-Rose Ungunmerr-Baumann), a Daly River artist, notes: "The Australian continent is crisscrossed with the tracts of the Dreaming: walking, slithering, crawling, flying, chasing, hunting, dying, giving birth, performing rituals, establishing things in their own places, the landforms and water, making relationships between one place and another, changing languages, changing songs, changing skin" (quoted in Atkinson 2002, 35–36).

What results when the mythology, the spiritual culture of a people is lost, when people are dislocated from their culture, community and their earth place? That sense of the sacred in which meaning is symbolized and embedded, is thingified, and the loss of ritual and boundaries result in either a dead center which we call an autistic core, or a breakdown where that core does not hold, which results in the enactment of severe pathology and criminality.

## BEFORE AND AFTER THE LOSS OF A CULTURAL AND SPIRITUAL BASE

We can begin to explore the consequences of that loss of the sacred with the aid of two narratives. The first details the Djarada ceremony, and provides an example of Aboriginal spiritual culture in its intact state. The second, Kirra's narrative, depicts loss of spiritual and cultural meaning.

### The Djarada Ceremony

The Aboriginal people believed that when the Moon Man was on Earth, he was a great lover of women. He made many songs to make them fall in love with him. He made the big sacred ceremony of Djarada and gave it to us, so that a man could sing a woman to be his wife.

In her book *Australian Dreaming* (2005), Jennifer Isaacs tells the story of such a ceremony that may still be practiced today in remote areas. When a man sees a woman he would like to have, all his close male relatives help him. They go out into the bush, and create a sacred piece of ground with a big circle. In the center is an oval shape painted on the ground with red ochre and white pipe clay. It has a red center. This represents the woman's vagina. A tall pole is stuck in the ground just in front of the oval, and the pole is decorated with paint and feathers. This represents the male penis, and strings covered with white bird dung are hung from the top of the pole to represent the seminal flow. The men decorate their bodies with red and white paint and ochre bird dung.

When everything is ready, the Djarada man stands before the feathered pole with legs spread, knees bent, and hands on thighs. His grandfather and uncle kneel at the side and they begin singing the circle of love songs. They sway their hips back and forth in the rhythmic motions of lovemaking. In the first song, the dream is that the man will be strong and attractive to the woman he has chosen. In the second, the dream is that she will think sweet things of him in her own dreaming, and the dream in the third song is that she will dream of making love to him. Then he sings a fourth song to make himself more attractive to her; he rubs juice from the roots of a special bush over his body. He sings all day and all the next night, repeating the song cycle over and over. These songs never fail, and the woman can't help falling in love with the singer even if she didn't like him before. This story from Isaacs's book is also told orally and in other writings.

## KIRRA'S NARRATIVE: THE LOSS OF CEREMONY, THE LOSS OF MEANING, THE RESULT OF TRAUMA

Presented now is a narrative told by a young Aboriginal woman, Kirra, late in the first year of her therapy. The narrative is as Kirra spoke in a taped interview with me, and the incoherence is true to her speech:

> I'd been down at the pub with my girlfriends and my cousin Kylie. They seemed to be having a good time, but I was bored and I wanted to go home. I had never been with a bloke, and I had no thought of being with one at that time.
>
> On the way home Anthony Crowl was coming along the road behind me. I knew he was a "bad" one, and I was very uncomfortable about the way he seemed to be following me. Next, he gets close enough and he drags me down the passageway between the buildings. I try to scream; he puts his hand over my mouth, and he rips off my pants as he puts his hand up between my legs. I scream again and he bashes my head really hard against the bricks. My mouth starts to bleed, my jaw is broken. I hear a crack.
>
> I can't see from two black eyes from the bang against the bricks. Only that my cousin saw my shoe sticking out from behind the building, he [Anthony Crowl] could have killed me, because I knew who he was and that mean jail. My cousin yelled for help and dragged him off me. I don't remember anything else. I woke up in hospital two days later. My mum was sitting by the bed. You wanna know what she said? She said, "Daughter you been raped. It's okay because we gonna get a lot of money from this." There I was nearly dying; she was thinking about money for drugs. She pinched my jacket while I was unconscious. It was a beaut leather jacket I bought with my first pay that day. She took my wages out of the pocket. I was so low I didn't care. I just went home. After, when I said, "Hey I want my jacket back," [she said] "Love! I was bursting to do a pee, so I got

down in the gutter outside the Cop Shop in Botany Road where I was tellin' 'em about Anthony Crowl doin' you, and I got pee all over the jacket. It ain't any good anymore." (Excerpt from research interview, 2002)

What happened between those two narratives, the first full of meaning, ritual, culture, the second stripped of meaning, culture, and ritual?

## ABSENCE AND LOSS

Absence and loss are central to Aboriginal people's loss of land, family, community, spirituality and culture. The emotional loss of her mother through early abandonment played an important part in Kirra's story. It explains why we so often fail in our therapeutic work with these young women. The basic loss is re-experienced and the pain unbearable. "To be born Aboriginal is to be born into an ongoing, unfolding catastrophe. For each individual the disorientation is particularly awful because they have no way to process that catastrophe. Their culture and identity no longer give a sense of who they are or who they could become" (Jeff Eaton, personal communication to author, March 2011).

Bion (1977, 20) wrote, "The patient feels the pain of an absence of fulfilment of his desires. The absent fulfilment is felt as a 'nothing,'" He added, "Non-existence becomes an object that is immensely hostile and filled with murderous envy towards the quality or function of existence, wherever it is to be found." Could this help make sense of the suicides so prevalent in Aboriginal groups? If so, it would also make sense of the assaults that are so prevalent, of domestic violence. But when a certain threshold is crossed, this destructiveness is total—it is despair, in which there is not only a sense of being destroyed but of having no hope of finding life again, or of self ever being reconstituted. Is this what happened to Kirra? Bion (1977, 21). spoke of "the awful superego, so cruel, so powerful, so destructive, that it denudes [the self] of any right or will to live."

Michael Eigen describes it this way:

> We may or may not know all the details about our annihilated selves. But we know such things exist, even if we don't know what to say of them. Annihilation processes are part of the way we are constituted. We live with dead areas. My hope is that making room for our annihilated self will enable us to be less destructive. We often injure, even destroy each other, in order to reach the realness of our annihilated beings. How much destructiveness aims at "showing" how destroyed we feel? Therapy is one place to try to contact the annihilated self without destroying ourselves. Speaking, sensing, and imagining is a

less costly method of discovery than giving in to the compulsion to destroy. (Eigen 2006, 28)

As Kirra's therapy progressed, she began complaining of a terrible pain in her stomach. It became worse and moved further up towards her chest with each session. She told about other traumas. She told how her Aboriginal mother had left her with a strict but caring Irish grandmother at the age of three. How in adolescence she had gone looking for her mother and was so excited to find her in a squat in Redfern [inner-city Sydney]. She told how the mother wooed her with ideas of the two of them living together until her mother took her money, then threw her out abusively so she could go to buy drugs. She told how she swore she would never return, yet a few weeks later, the desperate pain to find her mother returned. She spoke of the pain of being lied to, and betrayed, but also of being so desperate she had to go with it.

Then she stopped going to work, and stopped coming to therapy. She called a year later; she was on drugs and wanted all the receipts from her therapy so she could claim it in her tax return. She arranged to pick them up the next morning. She never came. She had lost her job and her boyfriend; she said she was now fat and misshapen, and the therapist would get a shock when she saw her. Was once a week not enough to hold her against the tide of pain? Perhaps she was already set on that other road of self-destruction when she came to therapy. It was hard to understand why the local doctor was continually writing scripts for medicines and sickness forms for her to miss work. The force to numb the pain was greater than her motivation for recovery.

The whole process of attachment is lost through the generational gap. A person whose internal protection is lost is psychically experienced by the other as a "no person," and to the perverted, such people present as available victims to be treated as objects for use and abuse. The transgenerational tragedy continues. Many Aboriginal children are sexually abused in early infancy. In some communities, reports state that up to two-thirds of children do not reach puberty unmolested. The predator at some level senses the prey as having no internal protection. The schizophrenic terror of disintegration of the ego from persecution by bad internal objects is a reality in external life for many Aboriginal people.

## Loss of Self

Central to trauma is a deadened and deadening internal mother. The internalized good mother's containing womb was shattered. The internal holding psychic womb becomes a sterile womb that deadens all emotion. That which holds the unknown and unknowable "core self" part of us is violated and ruptured in a horrifying way—the fetal self is aborted. The central core becomes a "non-person." The sense of self is fragmented like a fetus being suctioned out in parts in an abortion. Negative fears are greater than positive hopes. There is no creative space. The inner world becomes a dark, frightening abyss instead of a safe and protective place. Life is rooted in abject fear and terror, freezing all emotion and joy in living. Sometimes, bits of emotional breakthroughs present in the form of flashbacks or dark daydreaming, or in nightmares. For a subjugated people killed like animals, children taken from their mothers from birth, all this is passed on to the next generation, with terrible consequences. It is passed on "because the mother, not having her own core self, cannot hold the child in a way that sustains the child's core self" (LaMothe 2006, 450).

## DADIRRI PERVERTED

At the local park on a Saturday night there will be a dozen Aboriginals sitting in a circle. They seem to have Dadirri in mind, but this is not the traditional sacred Dadirri circle where all pain is shared and held and transformed by the care of the others. They drink until Sunday night or until the police come, whichever is first. Some do drugs as well. Pain is not suffered. Pain is numbed—too many have suffered too much already. This is what happens when people lose that which is meaningful and sacred to them. Men neglect their partners, they leave, they are absent during a pregnancy, and they move through a nightmare world of drugs and petrol sniffing that does not give true dreaming but is better than the nightmare that reality has become.

It seems possible that the nightmare the men create for themselves has something in it akin to murder. That possibility is evident in the narrative told by an elder named Lirra. You will hear how, in Lirra's mind, loss from death, suicide, murder, sexual abuse, being taken by social services, and miscarriage are all seen as part of the same events. There is a mix of death, mourning, loss, suicide, murder, miscarriage, spirituality, and evil.

Lirra calls me the day of a family funeral—a suicide, the second in six months. "Where are all the men gone?" she asks. The answer is they are hiding in shame, numbed by drugs and alcohol—two suicides in one family, six months apart and at exactly the same place in the same dark lane. She talks and cries for an hour on the phone. The therapist cannot hang up. She lets her cry; she must hold her pain. Lirra tries at first to escape the truth, saying, "Foul play at hand and I will get those murderers who gave him the drugs." She finishes by saying, sadly now, and quietly resigned, "He is his own murderer. Why?" She comes to a session of therapy.

Later when she arrives, she begins, "Like something inside me froze—I froze." Then she starts to speak very fast, as if overwhelmed, and her narrative becomes free-associating, and hard to understand because of the speed. This is an extract from the transcript of the session:

> When my little girl was abused, I had to switch off or I would go down; I tell her now, if she goes down, she will take me down with her. [Her little girl is now a mother with four children, each by a different man; each has abandoned her. The time is all tangled up as if it is right now.] It's killing me, but I am saved because I have faith—the dear Lord works in mysterious ways. Bill died down the block in the lane at the back of Edward Street. You have to lift layers, pull back the blankets to see what is underneath. He was no saint, but he never deserved how she cornered him for one attack of DV [domestic violence].
>
> He was up there for this funeral, and they had a wake and he was so drunk, and he had this young woman and he had conked out from the grog with her. She must have got up out of the bed where they were lying and went partying. He woke up and went to wake her up and there she was on the floor. He thought she fell out of bed because she was drunk, and then he found she was dead. She had been stabbed and they had wiped her and cleaned her up, and then brought her in and put her near the bed. They even washed her, because the blood and stuff you can find [with] the florescent light they use. They couldn't find anything. Of course, they blamed him. Any "Abo" would do. He done himself in, killed himself in Redfern Lane the police reckoned, but we didn't believe it. Maybe they killed him, who knows.
>
> Then six months later there was Charlie, this handsome man. He was my mum's sister's boy. He came to Sydney, bless him, because he needed his family. He worked at the Annan reconciliation garden bridge, and he slept in a room in the pub there. He must have come to Redfern to see his family—a man found him lying unconscious on the ground. They rushed him to hospital, and we all went to hospital to see him. They turned off the life support on his birthday. [Her face is ashen, her voice quivers. You cannot help but see years of wear and pain on her face, weather-beaten.] It was just six months before our nephew Lizzy's son died in exactly the same spot and they reckoned he killed himself too. This week's been so bad. Out of the blue Jeannie died. Bill her husband had his heart attack. I was with him and then I was going to see Cathy, and Rob died, so I had to go to his funeral. I got back and got Louleine [her granddaughter who lives with her] and I was going to take her and go and see Cathy, and I get a call—Cathy is dead.
>
> Strange about Charlie, [when] they found him in the laneway there was a suspicious hit on the head, could have been from the fall the police said, and they just were not interested. They said he killed himself, he died of an overdose. That is strange because none of us even knew he took drugs. His girlfriend was pregnant. Would you kill yourself while your girlfriend was pregnant? She freaked out completely.
>
> Aunty Judy, she was another one. She was in Cootamundra Girls Home. See, my grandmother had abscesses on her legs and couldn't walk, so when my aunt and her husband split, the children were taken, the boys to Kinsella and Aunty

> Judy to Cootamundra. She was abused there, and she attacked the matron, in fact she nearly killed her, and she ended up in Parramatta Girls Home, didn't she? She was such a beautiful woman, but from there she began the self-destruction. She had a razor, and she would cut and cut at herself. Her face was so cut it was just a heap of scars, and the same for her arms and hands. No clean flesh left anywhere. Then she killed herself and they came and took baby Colin. A white woman came, and grandma was sittin' in a rockin' chair on the veranda and she just wrapped him up, this white woman, and she took him out of her arms. I can still remember the tears rolling down her cheeks. We never saw him again, but I always wondered what happened to baby Colin. When I was working in legal aid, I decided to find him. I found him alright: he was in Lithgow jail. Too late I was, he had just become another death in custody. He had been fostered with a family in North Sydney in 1975. We got baby Colin alright. We brought him back home too, but in a wooden coffin. We buried him. So many tragic meaningless deaths. (Excerpt from research interview. Transcript of taped material, given with approval of subject)

As I listen to Lirra's story, I feel as if I am somewhere I should not be. I have done something I should not have done. I will stand accused, and all good things and all good people will desert me. Bad will happen to me. It feels as if I am in the presence of something catching, contaminating, something that is touching an area inside my psyche I have not touched before; guilt, yes, but worse—a total disbelief in forgiveness and atonement for a sin I have not committed. I have opened Pandora's box, and I cannot get away from the terrible black things inside.

Time and time again I tell myself I am not affected by the lives these people narrate to me, and time and time again I have an outburst in another area of my life that I know is from the result of material that I have not processed, cannot process. I wonder how can they process it. The dynamic of regression and progression for a people who dare not, cannot, struggle to be born as a result of a core fetal terror, matches so much of what I am writing and thinking.

For many Aboriginal people, "the relation to the primary good object is one of a fear-enforced infantile dependence that is experienced as being smothered. . . . This explains why so many—80 percent—of young Aboriginals who commit suicide do so by a slow smothering, wrongly called hanging. For them, a good internal object involves the fear of the loss of their active ego by imprisonment in smothering passivity" (Guntrip 1968, 82–85). In the light of Guntrip's theory, one sees these adolescents or young men who commit suicide in custody as actively reversing out of life, instead of carrying themselves into it. The suicide rate is seven times the Australian average. Deaths in custody are an accepted phenomenon. Our jailed Aboriginal people are seven times the number of the rest of the population, and yet represent only 3 percent of the population. A whole race immobilized by fear—the frozen immovable state observed in many Aboriginal men and women who are not always actively suicidal but living dead in their psyches. One sees it over and over in the blank stares, the unseeing eyes, as if one were speaking to someone else, and in that far-off, autistic-like, vacant look, as if they are somewhere else. Even if Aboriginal people appear animated, there is an unreal, cut-off quality to their narrative. They are in a traumatized state. Behind the deadness lies a primitive, passionate aliveness too catastrophic to be experienced. The trauma, which was at the time too terrible to process, has been repressed in its raw primitive state. Terror is at the center of the shutdown (Tracey 2007).

## A YOUNG ABORIGINAL GIRL'S DREAM

Martha is fifteen years of age when I first meet her. She was fostered at age five to an Aboriginal family. Even at that early age, she was already prone to self-harm and to attacking her foster parents and members of their family. She had no speech and became violent when frustrated in any way. The biological mother was and is diagnosed as paranoid schizophrenic. Drugs and alcohol play a large part in this. The biological mother has access to her daughter but rejects this right. Martha's father is unknown to her; he could be any Aboriginal man wandering the streets of the inner city. The foster mother is angry, and every day finds it harder to cope. She has diabetes and high blood pressure, and is constantly exhausted. Martha is diagnosed as mildly retarded and traumatized.

Martha is in year nine now in a special class. She can read and write certain words, but is limited in any real formal learning. In the last two years, since the age of thirteen, Martha has become intensely rebellious. A boy at school teased her. Martha raced out and sat in the middle of the road with the traffic swerving around her. Her lack of awareness of danger in her real life is frightening. She describes her biological mother to me:

> Her face looked like stone, she looked poor and sick. She can't give me anything because she needs all her money to buy food. Don't want to see her anymore. I want to catch a bus and go anywhere. I will never be able to work because I am dumb and slow in the head, and I can't read. I'm no good at any stuff! I hate school, I hate all teachers. I hate it because I'm no good at it. (Excerpt from transcribed interview)

She brightens up, saying, "I can play any sports though! I'm really good at sports. I'm very good at soccer, swimming, running, and football." Then her smile fades as she says, "I lose the words I want to say, and everyone picks on me because of that. You know I lose the words in my head. I'm dumb so I'm not any good." She asks me, "You some sort of a psych person?" "Sort of," I ask, "Why?" "Because I have this dream!"

Every night Martha has the same dream, sometimes twice. She is being chased, by whom or what she does not know, but it is terrifying and there are many pursuers. She reaches the edge of a cliff; she realizes there is nowhere else to go and throws herself over the cliff. She looks down and sees her body smashed on the rocks below. She knows that she is dead.

This is exactly what the colonists did when they settled in Australia. It was a kind of Sunday sport. A group of men would go out and chase a group of Aboriginals until they had nowhere to flee except over a cliff, where they would throw themselves off and die. This was an easy way of ridding the area of what they could only see as "vermin." Asked if she had heard that story before, Martha looked blank and had no idea. Is she living out her mother's madness? She is neither psychotic nor stupid. She is traumatized. Night after night she experiences and repeats the murder of her soul. It is a nightmare in search of an audience who can help her find meaning in the terror. Who inside her has written this "dream"? Who is the scriptwriter? Who is the director of this drama?

I do not dream hopeful dreams for Martha, but I cannot get her out of my mind. She haunts me day and night. I had very little feeling while with her. I experienced a state of mind like a concreteness of affect, a lack of anything one could hold. Perhaps I had taken on Martha's numbness. This is the incredible "non-person" quality that comes from transgenerational trauma. Her hopelessness stays with me. I keep telling her story over and over to my colleagues.

Three years later, I pick her up from the needle exchange bus. Martha is pregnant and much changed. She told me she was really great now that she was having a baby. Her foster aunt also told me that having the baby had saved Martha and she was doing just fine. Suffering of the suffering. With schizoid and autistic states, a new and different space is created that blocks any movement to and from the original space. The schizoid, autistic or narcissistic defense is a perversion of the real chaos, and only by release from this can movement to the abyss occur, and from that, a new beginning. In therapy or deeply moving life experiences, there is a freeing from this block to allow an inward journey to the core nothingness, where something may, but only may, begin.

Meg Harris Williams (2010, 26) says of Bion that, in his view "there is no pain without imagination, and, in the absence of pain, no mental life. There is instead a 'nothingness' for which many types of activity may be a 'cover.'" Later she adds, "[Bion's] writings are imbued with a sense of danger regarding the very real possibility that mental life can be extinguished if imagination is not, at the very least, 'given an airing'" (Williams 2010, 36). I write here of a particular kind of patient "who experiences the pain but not the suffering." Bion (1977, 19) said, "They may be suffering in the eyes of the analyst because the analyst can, and indeed must suffer. The intensity of the patient's pain contributes to his fear of suffering pain. He might even think he is suffering it because he mistakes feeling for suffering. For him, frustration and intense pain are equated."

The nature of the catastrophe for the Aboriginal people is that they have lost the cultural dreaming or processes that create the capacity to make meaning, and are left without a culture that gives a boundary to suffer it. They have the pain, but they cannot suffer it. Australia's first people have lost their scream, and with it their capacity to have their identity, which they now seek but which comes out in many destructive ways. "That scream is the birth from out of the autistic shell" (Jeff Eaton, personal communication to author, March 2011). Eaton, in his essay "The Obstructive Object" (2011, 17), writes, "According to Bion, some patients give evidence of living with an internal object that is ego destructive. Bion names this ego-destructive internal object an obstructive object."

Eaton puts the infant's scream, or failure to be able to scream, at the center. If that scream can be held in the mind of another, it is not evacuated violently into an action of self-destruction. It can be held, modified, neutralized, and contained. This is the central missing function for the young Aboriginal who kills himself.

## THE HEALING OF DADIRRI

Dadirri is a ritual that is found in every Aboriginal group, although it is known by different names, and it embodies the most ancient and most important form of healing. In Dadirri, the scream is allowed and heard, although it may not present as an actual scream. The elders gather around the traumatized troubled one and listen for hours in deep silence while the traumatized person talks and talks (this is his scream). It is the opposite of "thingifying." As Rose Ungunmerr explains:

> We sit in a circle around the person. We hear, in the depth of our inner spring. We do not talk, we own his story, his pain. The owning makes us one with him, it heals. This is Dadirri. A big part of Dadirri is listening. Throughout the years, we have listened to our stories. They are told over and over, as the seasons go by. When a relation dies, we wait a long time in sorrow. We own our grief, we

> share our grief, our group owns our grief and their owning of it allows it to heal slowly. (Ungunmerr quoted in Atkinson 2002, 136)

Dadirri transposes to the living situation of the therapy room. The therapist does not only talk; the therapist listens. By listening in depth, the therapist is witness to pain in a special way, enabling patients to express, to be, to speak from within their own culture. The therapist works with patients to restore a primary sense of meaning to them, to give a sense of value to the patients' primary way of doing and being. This is Dadirri.

In therapy, the deadened area becomes a space where agony previously avoided is tolerated, despair held, psychic pain of loss suffered, and fear contained. Awareness of dosage and timing are all relevant too. Interpretations that focus on love and hate or good and evil in the patient can be persecutory. The focus of psychoanalytic therapy needs to be on archaic denial and the fear, sometimes terror, of "knowing." Psychic holding is the main therapist–patient interaction. If internal holding is no longer adequate because of the intensity of the trauma, external holding is necessary for its resolution.

## CONCLUSION

This narrative fits well with Tustin's (1981, 191) concept of at-oneness. More particularly, it fits well with the idea that, in contrast to the nightmare that results from at-oneness's rupture, its presence leads to an overflowing of ecstasy.

Barinya is a rehabilitation unit for serious alcohol and drug users, located in a coastal country town. It is for people of Aboriginal descent. A village-like, live-in complex, it has a treatment center where people move from one therapeutic group to another throughout the day (Dadirri), eat nourishing food, engage in lots of physical sport and activity, and thus develop a different lifestyle. A young man from this rehabilitation unit speaks in one of the therapeutic sessions, at which I am present but not known. He is about twenty-years years of age.

> I have never been free of alcohol and drugs since I was 12 years of age. I have had a stormy past where I never worked and did all sorts of things to get drugs. I stole, I begged, I sold myself sexually. I have been clean for six weeks now. I can tell you it has not been easy. I am taking each day at a time. It is a nightmare, and I did not think I could do it, but it is getting better now. This morning I went in the bus to Smokey Cape lighthouse. From the green hill I saw the sun rising over the ocean. I felt something peaceful inside me, a kind of beautiful feeling of belonging as part of what I was seeing. I knew this was what I had been trying to find through taking drugs. I have been looking for this space all the time, but

drugs and alcohol didn't give me this space. They gave me numbness, no life. I do not know how long it will last or if I will have it again, but I know I have had this feeling and I will always know I have had it. (Except from therapy session)

## ACKNOWLEDGMENT

Reprinted by permission from Springer Nature: Springer Nature, Psychoanalysis, Culture and Society, "The autistic core in Aboriginal trauma: Breaking down or breaking out of the autistic defence," Norma Tracey, © 2012.

I wish to acknowledge the professional workers at Gunawirra and more recently at "Strong Mothers." Mike Eigen's mentoring and support have been important over many years. Supervisory discussions with Jeff Eaton from Seattle over twenty years has helped develop and continue to challenge the thinking out of which this chapter has been developed.

## *Chapter 9*

# From Oblivion to Being

## *Faith and Catastrophe*

What processes take place in a psychic move from oblivion to becoming, as the human psyche traverses from nothing to something? How do these processes create, impede, or destroy psychic birth? Thinking about these awesome questions opens up some exciting areas. Meister Eckhart (1981), Nietzsche (1969), Heidegger (1982), Bion (1977), and, in the real present, Caputo (1987) and Eigen (1993, 2004a, 2004b), inform the thinking here. In this earliest of all psychic events, there is a particular state of mind called paradox, for the mother with her infant in this very beginning of her infant's psychic birth as a person, and her psychic birth as mother to that infant. This chapter seeks to create a paradigm of what is repeated over and over in any therapeutic work with patients.

Faith is at the center and the question is what is the role of the mother in this faith? The mother is seen as the "holder of the faith," the father as the "protector of the faith." If she loses that faith, then she does not hold her infant in a way that allows the infant to remain in the suffering of the catastrophe. Her faith is not a belief in a good outcome, as indeed we see many mothers holding the faith with infants who they know will die. Survival is not a consideration. True faith sustains and holds regardless. This is perhaps the earliest idea of the mother as a container. Because central to the discussion here is the role of the mother in protecting and holding her infant regardless. In so doing she creates the first paradigm of how catastrophe can be faced with the central role of the therapist as the holder of the faith.

## DISRUPTION OF THINKING AS A WAY TOWARD NEW THOUGHT

Being and not being, faith and no-faith, are not only not contradictory but also essential to each other and informing of each other. Sometimes the line between is so blurred that what looks life-giving is destructive, and what looks destructive is essential to psychic birth. That which is most valuable is also to be seen as that which is capable of most perversion and destruction. That which looks most harmful, such as the suffering in catastrophe that we seek to avoid most, is where may be found the very core of being and source of life. That which may appear most helpful carries in it the impeding of life, the destruction of possible birth. To add to the consternation, all these are in constant flux, since every apparently creative interpretation given at the wrong time or in the wrong dosage, becomes destructive and even poisonous. What is right today may be very wrong tomorrow. Just when the therapist has decided they truly know what is going on and where they are, flowing with the flux means they might just have had a glimpse and are in the dark and groping again. Who among us in the clinical setting does not become afraid, embarrassed, and ashamed of a cry that has come straight from the core being, that seems to lack both professionalism and careful thought, that even seems an "acting out" on the therapist's part only to find that this has been the most invaluably useful shared experience in the whole therapy? How often too does a patient view the very worst nightmare of their life coming to pass in such a way that a new light and meaning and purpose is given to their life? "You've destroyed my map," one patient yelled at me, "and now I realize you don't have one either, the whole of this therapy business is a con. You tore up the only map I had, and you're as lost as I am!" The therapist does not make the rules, but does obey them, as hard as it is too when everything seems to want to pull in the opposite direction, not only from the patient but also from the whole flow of life. Only with some processing can the patient's very words of blame tell the therapist they are on the right track. The same happens with another patient, who is bitterly recriminating. "You know what you've done. You've reduced me to fuckin' ordinary, that's what you've done." Instead of the certitude of knowing, the therapist is left wondering, "Is he right; am I mucking him up?" It is only faith in the process that says this is how it needs to be if he is to be real and find himself.

> Meister Eckhart was the master of the disruption of thinking through and thinking against ordinary conceptions. If you think God is the master of being, he will tell you God is "pure nothing," without even a bit of being. If you took him at his word and called God "pure nothing," then he would show you God is "pure

being." The more anyone would talk about God, the more he would pray God to rid him of "God." (Caputo 1987, 268)

You don't have to be talking about God or be a mystic here to understand this. Caputo could just as well be talking about believing in psychoanalytic concepts.

A patient recently arrived for his session distressed and guilt-ridden. The day before, his very much loved seven-year-old son was overtired and refusing to have a sleep, and became so abusive towards his mother, that the patient "lost it." He grabbed the child, dragged him to his room, and finally, with some more provocation, walloped him. My first thoughts were, how amazing that this man acted spontaneously at all. Even his movements were measured and wooden, and he looked like he thought about each step as he took it. I grasped the moment and said it sounded "good" to me. He was astonished and even more astonished when that night he apologized to his son and his son said, "Dad, dad! It's OK! I had it coming!" They started to talk and ended up planning a three-day trip together, back to where he grew up, and then on to Ned Kelly Country. I tried to think about this trip later. They camped and fished in the same river he used to fish in as a small child. The "hiding" far from being damaging was like some rite of passage through to latency, and yet it looked so wrong. I was thinking about how Ned Kelly was a hero to some and a truly evil man to others, and how the good police were the corrupt guardians of the law in their pursuit of him. Interesting that he should be so important as part of Australia's mythology, this man who was so good and so wronged, or so wrong and so bad, and yet made out a hero.

It is in that state of mind where one doesn't know, where one is prepared to be in paradox and flow with the flux, that the best searching and thinking is done, as the patient I quoted above found, he would have to make a new map; a map having in it knowing and unknowing, believing and not believing. The very systems and concepts of psychoanalytic therapy are challenged and reconstructed with every patient, which leads to finding the movement from oblivion to being, and the meaning in psychotherapy of the return to catastrophic beginnings and beyond that to where there is the no-thing space.

"The catastrophic nature of its own life is the first and most basic task the psyche must take up" Eigen (1993, 214). Until one is psychically alive, one cannot know about the terror of annihilation, and yet the central core of being alive has to do with surviving the terror of annihilation. That beginning is like making a massive effort to pass through a force field, an anti-life field, where the "big bang" that destroys all is also the "big bang" out of which life is born. Hopefully, the result is the triumph of Freud's Eros over Thanatos, but not always, and that is why I want to also look at madness, and the price of real tragedy and trauma in our own later living experience. In the latest scientific theorizing, the "big bang" was followed by an immediate, incredibly speedy, and massive move of parts gathering together to survive. Eigen, through Bion, sees this early time as filled with "primordial terror." He says, "for Bion there is something terrifying in the very birth of self and the latter's inextricable tie to oblivion that is part of it and that it is part of" (Eigen 1993, 216).

It is that sense of catastrophe that links aspects of the personality.

> Cataclysm is a formative part of our being. . . . The first thoughts were non-thoughts. Objects compounded of things in themselves, feelings of depression, persecution and guilt, and therefore aspects of the personality linked by a sense of catastrophe. . . . [For Bion] first thoughts are catastrophic hallucinatory bits and pieces which seem to function chaotically, that is without reference to one another. In optimal growth this dispersed state culminates in the emergence of genuine coherence. (Eigen, 1993, 218).

The intensity of this terror, as bodily, mental and emotional states are fused, can be seen in earliest infant states—the scream in the scream. The transmuting of such primordial emotions to emotions that can be thought about and thought through, heralds the advent and the evolution of self (alpha elements). To achieve this awareness of catastrophe we must tolerate "fragmentation, whirls of bits and pieces of meaning, meaninglessness, chaotic blankness, dry periods, psychic distancing" (Eigen, 1993, 218).

In *The Electrified Tightrope* (1993), Eigen develops and extends the ideas of Bion, examining how Bion gave equal value to disintegrating as to integrating. "Bion tries to tap into a dimension in which it is an innate part of self's rhythm to fall apart and come together again" (Eigen 1993, 213). This giving of equal value to disintegration is a very important step. It takes away a sense of having "arrived at," for example, the depressive position. Eigen speaks of the "elemental and ubiquitous presence of the mind's ability to divide and unite" (1993, 213). This kind of thinking views our role as therapists very differently, and it becomes not the "arrival at" that is our goal; indeed, it frees us from having a goal, thus allowing the holding of our neutrality as we help the patient release that which is frozen in the dynamic between integration and disintegration, between catastrophe and faith.

Klein and Winnicott saw the depressive position as the goal to which we all aspire. The depressive position they saw as the place where the love and the hate meet, and were able to be identified within the one person. Here opposites could meet and become neutralized. The depressive position appeared as a goal to be aspired to, for here in a sense true guilt is born and a sense of reparation and symbolization could occur. They also gave it a developmental time frame. Bion saw this as an ongoing dynamic and emphasized the importance of disintegration as much as integration, for in disintegration was true self born again. The real sickness is not that the person has disintegrated, but that the holder of the faith has the capacity to wait for the disintegration, and to wait in the disintegration for integration to come. They hold the faith. It is interesting that in our language are phrases like "losing the faith." "he has the faith," "he is a true believer," "he does not believe anymore." These are all language around this issue.

Often the emotionally deadened patient is avoiding the experience of catastrophe and the terror of death. A patient of mine, when asked during a totally deadened and deadening of my session, whether he was suicidal replied, "No. Why would I need to kill myself? I am already dead." He did become suicidal later, but only when he began that first move towards life. Eigen (1993) and Bion (1977) write of the need for distance between us and the catastrophe, otherwise we are in it, and part of it, in such a way as there is no observer to know about it or think it. I want to give an example of this with the case of David, which I will then use to take us into the meaning of faith and its dynamic with, and meeting with, catastrophe.

## CASE: DAVID

The ward sister in the burns ward referred David's problem to me as the ward team coordinator. She said, "Yesterday, you were talking about babies, so traumatized when ill and missing their mother, that they despair and stop feeling. Look! I think I've got a baby like that here. He is lying staring into space like he's given up. The night sister said he has been like this for hours. I've called the rest of the ward team. Can you come?" We gathered around the bed—sister, surgeon, occupational therapist, physiotherapist, social worker, and me. The baby was unresponsive and unaware of our presence. His eyes were open, but he was not looking anywhere. His arms were tied to the side of the cot, as he had tried to scratch at his buttock burn in distress in the night before.

"We should get the mother in," we said. She lived in the next suburb. When the ward social worker telephoned saying her baby was missing her, she responded immediately. She had wanted to come but had another little one and no transport. We all agreed her little one could come to the ward. The social worker drove her in. A concerned mother arrived. On the way in, she talked about her guilt and feeling responsible for the accident. The physiotherapist put sterile gauze on mother's knee so David could be nursed by her, but he did not acknowledge her presence. She was nearly crying herself as he looked into space. The occupational therapist sat with them. David let out a little whimper, which became a continuous crying and whining, and eventually developed into a kind of wail. Sometime later, the sister telephoned me.

"Look! We are all going crazy down here. David hasn't stopped crying for a minute since you left. We have done the wrong thing here, and we have made him worse. We can't stand it." I came down. It was an intolerable cry, and neither the ward staff nor the mother could emotionally make sense of it. "We can't have done the right thing," the sister said. "We were supposed to make him feel better. We can't stand this." There was chocolate dripping from his mouth where his mother had tried to quieten him. The staff were jittery, and after a short time my own feeling was of being invaded with something intolerable. I telephoned my colleague friend. "Everyone is going crazy with this baby's crying," I said. "He is letting you all know how terrible it's been. He needs to cry!" he said. I spoke to the sister. "David is telling his mother how terrible it was without her, and until he does this, he can't emotionally find her." She went to the mother. "He wants you to know how terrible it has been." Mother nodded. Tension dissipated in the ward. Even junior nurses were saying "Poor little thing. He's telling us how awful it was."

In the following days, David's mother came all day and after work his father came too. David was difficult a lot of the time and expressive of his pain, but there was no longer a question of him not being emotionally in touch with his mother or the staff. The sister reported to the ward team: "We learnt a great deal from David. We now always admit the family with the burnt child. Even though it is a lot more work and emotional pain for us, we think tolerating the crying and disturbance on our ward is worthwhile."

## FAITH

I have narrated a simple ward event. Understanding what happened in David's inner world is more complex. If the mother is not there as the holder of the faith, there can be no faith, and no entry into catastrophe. What is faith and where does it come from? I learned from David where faith comes from. Faith is right at the core of the catastrophe. It is the cry of the infant, who if he did not believe the mother would hear him would not cry. David lost faith and closed down, and we now know this is a real physical event in the hippocampus, the amygdala. When David found his mother to cry to, he had faith he would be heard, and he could suffer the catastrophe in the catastrophe, the suffering in the suffering.

The baby who goes into a kind of detached stupor, as Bowlby classically describes, has no faith that he will be heard. I am always taken by the words in the Bible: "I cried out to the Lord, Lord hear me"; or "I cried out to the Lord, and he heard me." And if he does not hear: "To you Oh Lord I call: My rock hear me. If you do not heed I shall become like those in the grave" (Psalm 28).

If the infant is not heard, that infant has no faith. If he cannot go into catastrophe, because it is too terrible to go into without the "holding" of his mother, then he becomes numbed and deadened.

> If when we speak of the "eyes of faith" we do not mean that a special light shines on the believer, which is withheld from the rest of us, but rather that he has a certain faculty to construe the darkness, to grope in the dark. Such eyes are accustomed to the lack of evidence and to living without assurances. (Caputo 1987, 79)

What is the role of "the other," the mother in faith? The mother to me is the "holder of the faith." If she loses faith, then she does not hold her infant in a way that allows the infant to remain in the suffering of the catastrophe. True faith sustains the holding regardless—blind faith? Survival is not even a consideration. This has got to be the earliest idea of a container and in a way as Eigen describes it, "an infinite container." The role of the mother in protecting, holding, creates the first paradigm of how catastrophe can be faced with faith, and a beginning of psychic self-becoming. Her capacity to sustain her infant through the no-faith area of catastrophe means he will not have to prematurely foreclose, as occurs in numbing such as David's, and much more seriously in psychosis.

Initially, a mother is emotionally present for her baby because she has an emotional meaning for herself as mother, and she has faith in that meaning. There are, however, mothers for whom this faith is lost. I conceive that the problem of the depressed mother is that she has no faith that if she falls apart, she will come together again. As I noted in Chapter 6, I would further suggest that in some early stage in a depressed mother's life, her own mother, the "holder of the faith," has failed her and has failed to hold her through the catastrophe. She has proof in her past of disintegrating and of not coming together again. She is therefore frozen in terror and dares not go into catastrophe, so there is no resolution, no arrival at her own central core of being. The catastrophe then is either disassociated from in the way I describe in madness, or never recovered from and always present. The central core where rebirth takes place is continuously destroyed, so no birth can take place and in the place of life is deadness. The problem of the depressed mother may well be that she dares not go into the catastrophe and go "mad," and therefore cannot reach sanity. If we are to describe the role of the therapist, I would see it as unfreezing the tension or movement between faith and no faith, in a way that allows entry to the catastrophic and the core of being.

I shared a workshop with a priest colleague of mine whose task it was to debrief missionaries returning from serious war-torn areas. They had faced horrendous situations, risked death and disease, but seemed to have spiritual energy to meet the needs of those they served, even when they were abused for doing so. They seemed fine while they were there. When they came home to the motherhouse, they disintegrated, lost the meaning of who they were and questioned "why" they were doing what they were. In fact, they seemed to question not only the meaning of their lives, but the meaning of any life. Amazing stuff! Even the best and most sublimated actions calling to hold faith in the catastrophe of others, may be either a help or a hindrance to reaching our own catastrophic center. The missionaries needed to be safe in their motherhouse before it was safe to face their own inner turmoil.

## "THE GROUND OF THE SOUL": THE CENTRAL CORE

The central core of what we become is not only the province of psychoanalytic thinking. Philosophers had added much to the debate far before we became a profession. For the background to this thinking, I am indebted to John D. Caputo, author of *Radical Hermeneutics* (1987), and emeritus professor at Syracuse, where he taught after leaving Villanova University, Pennsylvania. I am amazed that the philosophers looking at radical hermeneutics are so in tune with our thinking here, and how Bion and Eigen were able to absorb this as part of analytic thinking. It is of the utmost relevance that we have discourse on this now. For it is where we return in our analytic work over and over again. Sometimes life takes us there as in the cases I present throughout this book, but always our work in the analytic encounter takes us to the dark night of the soul, to the point of deconstruction and reconstruction. Caputo (1987, 268) writes,

> Meister Eckhart said that beneath the busy work of conceptualizing and willing, down at the base of the soul there is a certain deep spot, which he called the "ground of the soul," where the soul is able to establish contact with God in a way which broke through all the *Gerede* or ordinary conceptions of God. "At that point," he said, "we have a sense not of being flooded with light, but of having fallen into an abyss (*Abgrund*) where all the familiar conceptions we have devised about God collapse."

Caputo goes on to say that Eckhart saw this as a breakthrough (*Durchbruch*), but at that point we get a sense of not being flooded with light but having fallen into an abyss (*Abgrund*). Although Caputo saw it as the place where God broke loose from the confines of our nonsense values of who God is, "all hell break loose in this space did."

> [It is] the moment of midnight reckoning where the ground gives way, and one also has the distinct sense of falling into the abyss. . . . It is found in Kierkegaard when he talks about fear and trembling, in Heidegger quite pervasively and in Derrida, and in Husserl, in the description of the annihilability of the world, its vulnerability in principle to decompose, deconstitute, deconstruct, leaving nothing behind but the pure time flux. Radical hermeneutics arise only at the point of breakdown, breakthrough, breaking out. In this space we confront the loss of meaning by confronting the meaning of loss. (Caputo 1987, 269)

This is not very different to what we are speaking of in our psychoanalytic encounter. Heidegger's notion of *aletheia* is relevant here: "That from which all things spring up and that to which all things return . . . It is nothing as safe as a rounded whole in which being clings to itself but a fluctuating play in which things are never reduced to what they are" (Heidegger 1982, 78). Heidegger used the word "unencompassable" (*Das Unumgängliche*), the thing (no-thing) we cannot get around and therefore cannot avoid running into. This is not just the absence but the play of presence and absence, the unsettled fluctuation between the two, so we can never lay hands on a fixed structure or a stable stuff (Caputo 1987, 270).

I want to look here at how close this thinking is to Eigen's thinking. In his book *The Psychotic Core*, Eigen writes:

> In a sense, faith fights catastrophe with catastrophe. It can shatter our attempts to cling to well-intentioned security systems. Contact with a catastrophic reality shatters the lies we have built up to protect ourselves. To blunt our awareness of catastrophe is to lose or never gain a sense of who we are. Faith thrives at our cutting edge. It sustains our approach to and our tolerance of our selves. It keeps our sensitivity to ourselves alive. Our personality deepens . . . If [the analyst's] sense is deeply rooted in the non-sense beyond knowing, his work may have a resonance that makes a difference. (Eigen 2004b, 138)

This kind of thinking is akin to Caputo's notion of flux. Caputo (1987) says without this notion of flux, faith becomes a dangerous dogmatism. Again, not very different to the idea of psychodynamic therapy, where our constant effort is to stay in the flux between two opposite pulls. Certainly, the same can be said of our thinking during the therapeutic process, and our thinking of what our institutions are really about. There is a dangerous antilife feeling around in some of our institutes; feelings of superiority, of being anointed with holy oil, with some analysts not mixing with the lesser species lest there be a danger of getting watered down or contaminated, of losing the ultimate purity of perfection of thought. There is a feeling that we are superior to other professions, or they cannot see things as clearly as we do. There is a feeling if we do short-term work, it is because we cannot cope with long-term work, that if we care about people while they are suffering in real-life situations, this is inferior to caring for them years later when the suffering has by this time festered and become dangerous to their existence. That working directly with mothers and fathers in the early days of pregnancy and birth is not half so exciting or valuable as dealing with the problems created by these going wrong some ten or twenty years later. "It may be psychoanalytically informed," one of my colleagues told me "but it is not psychoanalysis." It is sometimes as if the only pure work is that of the encounter from the analytic chair to the analytic couch, rather than seeing equal value in each work.

It is as if the world only began with psychoanalysis, and as if we have the one true faith, and the others are less fortunate souls who live life not in the light of truth as we do, but in the dark. Terrifying stuff! Stuff which will kill our institutions struggling as part of the beginning catastrophe to formulate themselves. We are in serious danger of rigidifying our faith, and in doing so, destroying the very thing we aim to create. We need to flow in the flux, not only in our work, but in our institutions, if we are to survive. I guess even the presenting of this, which we have all thought about in the recesses of our own minds but never dared speak, challenges the system out of which it is born, not to take life from it or to criticize it, but to liberate it.

> So if we speak with the eyes of faith, we do not believe that a special light shines on the believer which is withheld from the rest of us, but rather that he the believer has a certain facility to construe the darkness, to grope in the dark. Such eyes are accustomed to the lack of evidence and to living without assurances . . . The eyes of faith mean that the believer is good at making his way through the dark, at keeping on the track of the divine. Far from being able to see God everywhere, the believer has perhaps the sharpest sense of all of the withdrawal of God, His absence from the world. (Caputo 1987, 279)

Could this perhaps help us with where we are going? The space in our work with our patients leaves us so alone, and the absence of a guiding light of certainty in this space where as Bion (1977) says "we must be free of passion and memory and desire," leaves us so much grappling in the dark. Sometimes with the best will in the world and unknown to ourselves, we grasp at an interpretation prematurely, hoping to fill an unbearable space or to assure ourselves of our control of a situation for which we do not and cannot have control, where we do not and cannot have answers. The implications for my work are enormous. If I have any sense of certainty about any of my thinking with a patient, I freeze the movement and flow between us. I cannot ever afford the luxury of certainty with patients, especially if it is born as a defense against uncertainty. The relevance of being in the catastrophe with our patients is what I thank Eigen's work and writing for in my clinical work each day.

A state of mind akin to hallucination needs to be accessed if we are to be empathic and involved in the catastrophe. Not only is the new order born in chaos, but that order then becomes the old order, and it needs to collapse for another new order to begin. This ongoing dynamic is the name of living in the work. Believing God can hear us in the core of our suffering is faith, or even being aware that he cannot hear us, is faith too. There can be no greater terror than to think you have your "other" there in the catastrophe with you, and then to have the horrible realization you are alone. You do then fall out of the hands of the living God.

## CASE: MELANIE

Melanie has a healthy, full-term, thriving four-month-old male infant. She presented for therapy saying with the birth of her infant she had "lost herself" and was continuously crying and distressed. Her mother and father had come from Canada to Australia for the birth of the child. During their four-month visit she was horrified to see her mother "kind of like losing her mind." Every day she would ask the same things, like, "Where did you say the spoons were, which drawer?" I commented she felt she had lost her identity, and she was here telling me of her mother who also seemed lost. She said she felt guilty, as if she should never have left her parents and married. She was aware that from the day she was born her mother was dependent on her. She felt it was her place to keep her mother alive. Now with her leaving home she had taken life from her mother. Her mother seemed dead or dying to her now, and it was all her fault. Through her childhood and until she left home, her parents had been totally involved and preoccupied with her swimming prowess. She has always been "driven" by them and herself, becoming a champion swimmer in her native country.

In the fourth session she said, "Everything you say makes sense. These are thoughts I have never used before, but you have really failed me because I came seeking advice and you haven't given me any. You have given me no sense of direction that I should go in. I would have thought any therapist could have done that." As her therapist, I experienced a strong pull to give her advice but knew such advice would be spurious and not from within herself. I told her this; it seemed to frustrate her more. She left and rang me that week to say she would not be returning. I worried about having failed her for days. Had I not been alive enough for her, I wondered. Later I began to think maybe I was carrying her feelings about having failed her mother. Such is the power of primitive projection; one can never be sure what one is carrying. Our discussion group was very divided. Some felt there was an empathic breakdown on my part, others said her leaving was a move toward health, wondering if she needed to fight with the mother and walk out on her to find herself via me.

In many of these cases, one is left without a feeling of resolution and often there is great difficulty in understanding what role one plays in the transference. I think there are reasons for this. One is that the transference is psychotic, in the sense of being "the thing in itself." This is not necessarily a sign of disturbance. I think it is an external living out of the characters of an internal drama awakened by becoming a mother, and the primitive emotional arena inhabited in this life stage. I think it is important to acknowledge this. There are mothers who with the birth of their infant are hurled back into some repressed trauma. Here they feel out of control of their emotions and behavior. They are at some early primitive mental and emotional level, where the way they think, feel, and act is internally dictated, not in their control or that of the therapist. Health professionals who are hoping through their work with these mothers to atone for or repair their own internal objects (by being a good mother to their patients) are not at all in the right frame of mind to do this work. I am often left months later wondering what went wrong. Why did I act as I did? Did I do good or bad, or even nothing?

I think this case illustrates how old conflict is reawakened by the birth of a baby, particularly conflict to do with separating out from the mother. In such cases internal events, often requiring years to uncover in therapy, present themselves as the earliest crisis repeats. In the end, as in any therapy, our presence and the creating of a psychic space might provide the space to do the work which could not be done before. Sadly, sometimes it is not the resolution of that past but a repeating of it, and often the therapist may feel helpless in this. There is often a feeling of being in catastrophe, not of one's making or control. Some six weeks after she finished, a beautiful card arrived from Melanie. "Thank you," she wrote. Nothing else. Just "thank you."

## CASE: JOANNE

Joanne highlighted this even more for me. She is a mother in our mothers' group. It was a particularly cohesive group. They had met weekly during their pregnancies and were so involved that they were all back at the group within a few days of their births. One came back on the train, five days after the birth, and she had had a caesarian. Another got her husband to come and get her from her hospital bed and bring her to the group accompanied by her mother-in-law, and another brought in pictures of the whole birth and passed them around. These groups are described as a space in which mothers can think about their role as parents to their infants and partners, and with each other. The support they gave each other always extended into the community.

Joanne arrived at the group without a hair on her head out of place. That is the best way I can describe her. She was very high up in the computer industry, and extremely successful at her work. As I have described, this was an exceptionally close group, but Joanne seemed distant from it all, though she never missed a session. I heard "IVF" hinted at or muttered about at one stage. Joanne's baby, despite heroic efforts on her part, refused the breast, and so she expressed and fed from a bottle until he was five months old. But he would not touch the breast. The special consultant she had gone to see about the problem had said, "You've got Norma in the group. She is terrific! Have you talked to her about it?" Joanne said, "No, Norma is preoccupied with Marianne, her favorite. I don't think she is interested in me." The consultant reported this back to me and I was amazed. However, I did realize whenever I tried to communicate with Joanne there was this extraordinary gap between us, a gap I could not ever make any sense of. Joanne did not inspire the protective maternal warmth in me that the other mothers did.

When her baby was six months old, and he was a beautiful, thriving baby, Joanne was away from the group for three weeks. When she returned, she told us about her trip to her parents in another state. The women were all talking about would they or would they not get pregnant again and when. One of the mothers made the remark to Joanne that she would probably get pregnant quicker next time, since the previous one had taken five years. She said "Well, it will be a virgin birth if I do." "You used donor sperm?" I spontaneously replied. How I regret that reply and how I regretted it for weeks afterward. Joanne sat there not answering, then a tear or two came, and then she burst into tears, and sobbing wildly, she ran with the baby from the room.

I signaled to one of the other mums, Di, who was her particular friend to go to her. Di went out and I could hear Joanne absolutely sobbing. I excused myself from the group and went to her. Joanne was in a blind rage and turned it all on me. "How could you ask such a question? No one knows except my husband and my mother! You've told everyone. How could you be so insensitive. You should know that is the one question you can never ask." She then told us amid tears how she had been for three weeks to visit her mother in Shepparton, and everyone in the town kept commenting on how much the baby was like his father, and no one knew except her and her mother that the baby was IVF donor sperm. "Don't you ever ask anyone that question. You don't know what it's like, you don't know what I have suffered." It was quite terrible. Finally, she calmed down enough to come in and I said, "Let me make you a cup of tea."

I made her a cup of tea, and I sat down beside her, and I could feel her rage towards me. "I'm sorry, it's nothing to do with anyone else in the group, only you," she said, glaring at me. "I've got to leave." And she left. It was time for the group to break up, but they were very generous toward me, saying "Are you alright, everyone has been looking after Joanne, but are you alright?" I said, "No, I'm OK, but I can't believe I was that incredibly insensitive."

Strangely when I went out, I found Joanne still in the car park. I went over to her and she started again, "You don't know what I suffered." I said, "Joanne it was very hard to know you were suffering, you are always so together, so made up, never a hair out of place, always looking so self-assured." She said, "How do you think it feels to put that on every day for five years while your heart is breaking? Did you know that was my eighteenth attempt at getting pregnant? Eighteen sperm at $7,000 a sperm. Do you know what it is like to be told your husband has no sperm, do you know what it is like?" And all of this was with such accusation.

I went home feeling like death. I felt as if all the things that had ever happened to this woman I had caused. I knew this was not true, but I could not control the feeling inside me that it was. I rang one of my colleagues the next day and had lunch with her. Over lunch I shared the whole thing with her. I said to her. "How could I have been so terrible; how could I have been so insensitive?" She just looked at me and said, "I would have asked that question." This started to help me to come out of it. I stopped thinking "Do I ring her? If I ring her, I'm intruding. What do I do?"

That night she rang me. We talked on the phone for nearly an hour. She again shared with me all the things that had happened. She wanted me to promise I would never be a therapist to her. That was what I had done wrong that day, she said. I had been a therapist when she had really come to that group to have someone who was a group leader. Someone who was motherly was fine, but I had crossed the line and she did not know if she could ever trust me by coming to the group again. I told her how terribly sorry I was to have opened such pain for her, and I was thinking I never am nor ever will be as much a therapist as when I was there agreeing not to be a therapist again, holding her in on these assaults, which went on and on. She then told me, and I was horrified, how they had forced her to see a counselor, or she would not be allowed to use the donor sperm, and how she had reluctantly gone and felt that the counselor had been totally insensitive to her sense of shame that she had had to resort to this level to have a baby.

It was then I started to become aware that I was carrying the load for someone else, ridiculous that I couldn't see it before, but I was so much in it with her. The load became easier for both of us. She said she would return to the groups because she liked the mothers there, but I must never play therapist with her again.

I actually was starting to get understanding now. Professionals had crossed the line into her privacy, into her womb. A strange seed had been implanted there. This is mad making I thought. It was unbelievably hard for her and me in the groups together the next time, and indeed for weeks after. We were both in a black unbelievable depression. She spoke to everyone in the group except me. We both of us worked so hard to try and find each other, indeed I thought we would fail. I was ready to give up and planned to punch in the nose the next person who said, "but you are only doing supportive groups not analytic ones, aren't you?" But then let me share how it broke. Joanne was a singular mother who never encouraged her child Robbie to go to anyone else. One day in a very gingerly testing way she said, "Go to Norma, Robbie," and pushed him towards me. He came into my arms and she said to me, "Would you nurse him while I have a cup of tea?"

The following week, a fine-looking man arrived before her carrying all the bags and stuff. She followed carrying the baby. He put the stuff down and took the baby from her. He put his hand out and shook mine. "So you are dad," I said. "I am," he said. "I am the father of Robbie. I have heard so much about you." I asked Joanne later what he might have heard and she said, "he was so relieved that someone else was copping it, not him now, that he felt a real affinity with you."

Joanne improved a lot from this time and became a lot more human in the group I thought. Eventually she brought her mother to one of the groups. I felt that we were invaluable to Joanne. This was the one place in the world she could talk freely about the IVF. Every detail of implantation and the beginning pregnancy of the next lot, twins, was shared with the group week by week. When the twins' arrival was due in a few weeks, I sensed that Joanne was again having trouble talking to me. Indeed, she turned away and it became very obvious. I waited for this to result in something, maybe after the babies are born. I felt she still had a great deal of pain. I wished so much to help her, yet I knew in a way I cannot. She needed to go through it. She rarely missed a session. Two mothers in the other group were pregnant at the same time and had a real affinity with her. We combined the groups and this brought them together. I wondered about all the other IVF mothers in her situation in life, how do they get to work it through?

## SPACE

There are two "no-thing" spaces in Bion's work. They are at very opposite ends of the spectrum, and both Bion and Eigen write a considerable amount about them.

There is this nothing space born out of hatred of being, which destroys the meaning of things and robs them of their life. By doing this, they leave an empty space inside the person, a space where living would be if it could be lived. In "Transformations," Bion says,

> Space may be personified by a non-existent "person" whose hatred and envy is such that "it" is determined to remove and destroy every scrap of "existence" from any object, which might be considered to "have" any existence to remove. Such a non-existent object can be so terrifying that its existence is denied, leaving only the place "where it was" . . . The "nothing" place is even more terrifying because it has been denied further existence and denial of the existence of the place where it was, makes matters worse because now the "point," marking the position of "no-thing" cannot be located. In accordance with Kleinian theory, such an object can be within the personality of the therapist or the patient. (Bion 1965, 111)

In writing about trauma, I have many times referred to this as the autistic space, the numbed area where thought experience could be thought and processed, if it was thinkable. Tustin (1981) saw autistic states as being preceded by a blinding rage.

The second type of no-thing space I do not think has to do with the first. Eigen (2004b, 45) speaks of it thus, "The 'is not' of no-thing that keeps the space open for development or for undoing development is, for Bion, a crucial psychological reality." This is the no-thing precursor of creative life—the space where old life can end, and new life begin. Eigen (2004b, 48) gives a meaning to the idea of "patient blankness or mute gestation." This is the no-thing space where waiting with the patient is of the utmost relevance. It is a twofold problem for us as therapists—that of being able to tolerate the nothing until the "something" from the patient is formulated, and in which we stay in the actual experience of the nothing. It would be wrong to ignore the incredible pull that comes from the patient to fill the no-thing. There can be little that is more destructive than precociously inserting our own thinking, our thing, into another's space. In doing this we destroy their thinking. In his book, *Psychic Deadness* (2004a, 47), Eigen writes, "The murder at stake includes the killing of mind, psyche, self and personality . . . [and as Bion] continues, 'Such procedures do not produce the results ordinarily achieved by thought, but contribute to states approximating to stupor, fear of stupor, hallucinosis, fear of hallucinosis, megalomania, and fear of megalomania'" (1965, 82).

I want to give a very simple example.

## CASE: CATHERINE

Catherine was referred in a most extraordinary way. After I left my local butcher shop with my meat, the butcher turned to the next customer, a man, and said, "There goes one hell of a smart little lady. That little lady works with people who are in trouble in their minds, and she helps them feel not depressed, you know OK about themselves." Some weeks later, this man went back to the butcher and got my address and came to my front door. He said, "Do you see depressed people?" I said, "Yes." He said, "Would you see my wife? She is very depressed," and I said, "If she wants to be seen." And he said, "My wife desperately wants to be seen, she sent me around to find you." "Well you let your wife call me" and I gave him my card. Hardly fifteen minutes passed, and a call came from her. I sent her to her doctor for a referral and she came. (A few weeks later I also got a referral for her husband for therapy.)

Catherine came with a sense that there was no hope she would ever find or even ever be allowed to have an existence of her own. She had never found it in her own home with her parents and now with her three children growing up, she was aware she would never find it in her marriage. And yet she could see no way out. I want to tell you a little story she told a vignette from her life; I must have returned to this 500 times over the time I saw her.

The mother and father came yearly from England to see her and her husband and children. They stayed for six weeks. Catherine always saw her mother to be invariably critical. When the little boys would fight with each other, the grandmother would say to her, "Your father and I are convinced those children are allergic to each other." The implication as Catherine experienced it was that it was something unfixable. But the incident that struck me most was a very small and simple one. I tried to share it with some colleagues and they failed to see the point of it. Some even saw what the grandmother did as harmless, and indicative of my patient's problem more than of any problem with the grandmother; perhaps if my patient was in a normal mother-daughter situation, it would have been all right, but because of the unknowing of the grandmother to her own daughter's feelings and the daughter's inability to express these, it was not all right, it was all wrong.

They had an old toilet brush in the bathroom. The brush had certainly seen better days; by the time it had been used over the years it had become very worn. Catherine's mother went shopping and bought a new toilet brush, and when she got home she threw the old one out and put the new toilet brush in the bathroom. She felt morally right and good about it. She and Catherine had words about it. Catherine saw her not as fulfilling a need she had for a new brush, but that her mother had seen the new brush as better and well chosen by herself, and in Catherine's mind had not considered her daughter's choice. The conversation went like this. "Where is my old toilet brush?" Catherine asked. "I threw it away," her mother said. "But I liked it." "Don't be ridiculous," her mother said, "it was totally worn out and I have bought you a vastly superior one . . . why are you never grateful?" "I would have liked to have chosen when to throw it out, and I would have liked to have bought my own brush."

Now what is so interesting about this story is that it mirrored almost everything in her life. Catherine never started a sentence that was not literally taken over by her husband, and his wiser and better thoughts and words substituted for her own. He actually did come from a family of preachers. She felt she was always wrong and any idea she had was inferior and meaningless, otherwise why substitute a better one. It is easy to see neither he nor her mother created a space for her to decide on, or even think out loud, and they substituted without her desire or leave. She could not develop or explore her own space.

Let me take you further into this story. When Catherine was three and a half, her third sibling was born. The parents planned on her sibling's birth that to ease the mother's burden Catherine would go to day care. She experienced this as being thrown out and her room made available for a better one as chosen by her mother and father. Each day her father took her protesting and screaming to nursery school on his shoulders, and later she just gave in, becoming mother's helper when she was at home. She was conforming and responsible, and her profession became running an agency created by herself to find work for others in her industry. Why have I told such a simple story? Because it is relevant to what I am writing about foreclosure that interrupts and disallows continuity and expression. I am writing about the need to tolerate space and to give space. I am writing about an envious destruction that cannot allow anything to exist except itself. The meaning of what the person gives is annihilated and indeed the person themselves are turned into a nothing or as Bion or Eigen say, is thingified. Catherine could not create space for herself as mother or for her own children after they were born. She said she was a failure as a mother, and brought in a nanny who would be a better support for the children. She worked in the room next door, doing her work and coming in to breast feed, and then returned back to work. She could not allow space for her own creations—the nanny did all the minding.

Here I am talking about three different things, when we hasten too quickly and do not allow the space for order to come out of the chaos of catastrophe, then we have lost our faith in the patient as a person, and in that person's capacity to find their own way of life and self and living. At the point when our interpretations are premature, we cut across the patient's being; we may even be substituting our better thinking for theirs and we may be thingifying the patient. We stop the meaning of that person to themselves to emerge.

The hardest thing throughout this therapy with Catherine was to resist the extraordinary unconscious pull to fill her space. Not only was it a gravitation pull to fill it, but I felt guilty that I did not, and was in terrible conflict that I had failed her expectations by not filling the space. And only some sort of faith and deep past paradigm of my own inner work with my analyst, and my training seemed to hold through just enough to tell me don't budge.

This case ended sadly. Catherine decided she would prefer to live alone with her now grown-up children coming and going, rather than stay with her husband. He had made massive gains in his own therapy, drinking less and working very successfully in his career. Her one constant complaint was that in an effort to exist he always wiped her out, denigrating any thought she had until she was a no-thing. Eventually they settled for living in the same house, each with their own space.

Eigen (2004a, 45) writes, "The temptation to fill in, to thingify, or otherwise to nullify 'no-thing' is ubiquitous. . . . [It can create] a certain rigidity, tied to a defective or embryonic mental apparatus." Eigen adds that "an analytic interpretation may kill or support the growth of experience, including the experience of violation and dying out of self" (2004a, 47).

The psychotic cannot stay in the catastrophe, but because he cannot stay in it, he cannot leave it. For the psychotic, the catastrophe continues underneath for it has not been dealt with. The psychotic, having destroyed the potential of birth and new life, is stuck in the deadness. This is so in a lesser way for the borderline and the neurotic. The illness of the psychotic is not the hallucination, but that he is cut off from the empathy with it. For the mad person there are no symbols, Bion says, for symbols are facts and facts are symbols.

The birth of self "evolves" and "dissolves" around a sense of catastrophe. To reach the central core of becoming, we need first to touch in on the nothing. This requires an internal tolerance born out of faith, a faith that holds regardless, a faith that means groping in the dark, never finding infinite truth, but believing in it always.

## ACKNOWLEDGMENT

"From Oblivion to Being: Faith and Catastrophe," Norma Tracey, *The Psychoanalytic Review,* Volume 94, Issue 2: April 2007. Reprinted with permission of Guilford Press.

# *Chapter 10*

# Precreative Space

In Aboriginal culture, going back maybe 50,000 years, the physical place where the young Aboriginal woman was pregnant and gave birth to her baby was sacred ground, always revered by her and her community. The young pregnant suburban Aboriginal woman of today must reclaim that place, but now, instead of being land, it is the space of her body, mind, and emotions. She needs to reclaim this space from alcohol, drugs, and violence and declare it once more a sacred place of holding life and giving birth—the sacred land of new beginnings—not only for her infants, but for herself and her community.

At the core of the personality is a particular psychic space, which I describe as the precreative, primordial abyss. It is the nothingness, nowhere space, enunciated in most religions as the primary black void. It precedes all creative psychic living, all ambivalence; it is "before is and is not." It is not a static space, for there is a dialectical movement to and from it in every living experience, as old patterns of being are surrendered to allow return to the abyss but paradoxically for the first time, and from that be born psychically anew. I propose this dynamic as a continuum from birth to death, from womb to tomb, and as an integral part of living experience in every moment of our lives. In the primordial precreative space is the potential of life, risk, surprise, fear, danger, along with the possibility of the joy of creativity.

This chapter is about two different psychic spaces. We call the first space precreative. It can become procreative when there is holding and therefore the possibility of having life in it. The second space has its roots in abject fear and terror, for there is no holding in it. This is the dark abyss resulting from unresolved trauma. Death becomes more active than life as it works to annihilate life; terror freezes all affect. There is no movement. We call this space autistic or schizoid or psychotic. In the beginning was the darkness, the void, then because the void was tolerated came the light, the spark. The tolerance of that void allows intercourse, an intersection of ideas, an intersection of emotions, resulting chaos, any intersection "before actualization." It belongs before all intersections, all meetings, all intercourse in every human thought at every time and on every occasion and at every level. There is, for all of us, the ever-present threat of premature grasping from without, whether it is an idea, or a way of life, or even a profession such as psychoanalysis. If the nothing space has not been first entered into and suffered, that false grasping will become the roots of fundamentalism or obsession, with an external strong belief that is threatened by any other thinking but its own. Behind it is the terror of annihilation that cannot allow the journey to the true "nothing" space. It clings and cannot allow release. Meister Eckhart's (2001) little prayer stays with us, "I pray God to rid me of God." This, of course, links to the fundamentalist as one who confuses the raft with the ocean, religion with God, one's own opinion with God's own word, our low selves with God. It is a form of idolatry (Caputo 2001, 268). I am saying this is what occurs when we cling to the raft and dare not dive into the ocean and allow the oceanic to formulate again into the womb of our minds. This precreative space is before transitional space as described by Winnicott. It may well be the precursor of transitional space, but it occurs before anything is, so is not transitional in that sense. It has similarity in that it is the original space into which dreaming may occur, the space where we sing ourselves into creation.

## THE SPACE IN THE MIND OF THE PARENT

Parents first hold this space in their unconscious minds. The empty space predates parental reverie. Parents hold the memory of a void before there is a container in which to dream the possibility of a child into existence. Initially, there is no fetus, no child, not even a dream of a child, but a potential space to dream into. It may be in this space that faith is necessary as one holds the potential for the infant. In therapy, the therapist is the "holder of the faith" for patients to dream themselves once more into being and become themselves anew, tolerating the terror of the risk of oblivion. Infants, children, adolescents, adults have the psychic equivalent of a "time and place before I was" to which they return over and over again, each time to become anew. The paradox remains that the journey is always alone but cannot occur without the presence of "the other," and the other holds the faith by that presence. It may well be the space about which Bion (1977) writes in much of his work; a space that has no memory or present or future desire, yet it is the optimal space to realize. So, in this chapter, I ask what psychic events intrude that obstruct us from being in that space or disallow it, or destroy the possibility of intersection before it actualizes, that make for autism, narcissism, and other illnesses, that fail to allow for a two-thought, two-person intercourse, so that a false beginning of creation or a terror blocking all creation occurs.

## THE RELEVANCE OF THE PRECREATIVE SPACE IN THERAPY

I propose that therapists need to occupy this space through release from their own memories and desires. This release in the therapist creates an interactive event allowing for release in the other, the patient. The therapist must not only have the capacity to allow this space, but must also help the patient to arrive at it, so that the receiving and registering of the patient's input can occur, and so that the patient is in a place or state able to be receptive to what the therapist gives emotionally and psychically.

> The next thought involves the "location" of this space. I believe that this space is neither only in the therapist nor only in the patient. It is something that exists between and develops for each of the two. The patient and the therapist bring to the therapeutic encounter a willingness to enter into the stream of a process that cannot be predicted. Therapists may have from personal experience a conception of a previously arrived at precreative space, and can hold this as a potential that patients might discover, but they do not know the patient's space nor their own entry to that part of themselves in relation to "this" particular patient. When both therapist and patient dare to risk, dare to be surprised, cooperation occurs at a deep unconscious level. The two minds create a third entity that amplifies the precreative space as a shared experience, and this is where real healing and creativity occur, in ways that are aesthetic and emotionally awesome; neither the therapist nor the patient can orchestrate this, only create conditions where it might be realized. We see the therapist as a scuba diver teaching the patient how to stay underwater, go deeper. But the therapist too is risking and is once more diving for the first time, and observing and being surprised by the many beautiful and terrifying and strange creatures that emerge in the undersea world of emotional life, for it is in the watery depth that the intuition of being transcends dualism and can be an existential ground where O can have the potential of a glimmer of being. (Jeff Eaton, personal correspondence to author, 2006)

## THE PRECREATIVE SPACE IN ABORIGINAL THOUGHT

This space is the ancient space in Aboriginal culture. The most ancient of all known mystical thinking, central to all dreaming, is the idea of gunewari, "seed power." Gunewari is the invisible seed of life-creating energy. In the Dreamtime, where the creation of the world is continually being sung into existence, the unknown invisible seed engenders the energy of new life (Atkinson 2002). For Aboriginal people, pregnancy and birth are among the most sacred and precious of events, but they are preceded by the spirit of the Dreaming. Then, for Aboriginal women, pregnancy and birth become part of something sacred, because it is the Dreaming, not the symbol of it, but the Dreaming itself. This is a dreaming that can never be killed, and that is greater than human and finite life can be. Dreamtime narratives born from the earth give a "now" to all creativeness. Theirs is a perception of a "now" of all creativeness against a backdrop which cannot be created and so can never be destroyed—the Dreaming.

The Dreaming: we dream. Our dreams are all important—without our dreams day and night we would have no meaning to our lives. The psychotic with this deadness is trapped in the dreams, and the dreams concretize as if they are real. There is a primary collapse of the privacy of self, which may be linked to Freud's idea of the death instinct. The desire to die may or may not be involved, but the desire to hide, to disappear, to fade into oblivion is a way of hanging onto life by playing dead.

I think that the best basis for the concept of dreaming comes from Barry Smith, a manager at Aboriginal Children's Services. He has agreed to my retelling this story. Here is his story:

> I have never shared this with a white man, but because you are my special friend, I want to share this with you, Norma. I only went to school until I was 14. Because I had 12 brothers and sisters and I had to work, so some of the younger ones could go to school. When I was nine years old the Welfare decided to take all of us children from our mother and I remember being locked up in a cell, my mother and all of us kids in the local jail in Wellington. My mother called all her friends, and they came in and cleaned up us kids and washed us and put clean clothes on us and the judge said, "These kids look cared for" so he denied the order for removal. I am going to share a secret with you no one else knows outside of black fellas. Here is our story. In the beginning, all the black fellas were the one tribe, one family, and they all lived in the middle of the desert and spread out like this. [Barry drew a picture of spokes radiating from the circle center.] And then the white fellas killed them off here and here and here. [He showed places where massacres had indeed occurred.] But what no one knows and I am sharing with you, see all these lines [pointing to the lines radiating from the center], they only killed the people; they couldn't kill the dreaming. So now you know what the secret is, the dreaming is all still there, and that is why we are going to always be a people, and no one can kill us off. You can't kill dreaming. Dreaming lives longer than people do! That is our secret. No one can kill the dreaming. (Barry Smith, personal communication with author, 1992)

I came home thinking, "That's right! You can't kill the dreaming." What a powerful thought. You can't kill the nightmare either, day and night the dreaming, both the joy and terror in the nightmare, go on even in waking time. Even after we are dead the dreaming goes on. From generation to generation the dreaming, the joy or the terror continues. You can't kill the dreaming; you can't kill the nightmare in the dreaming.

## FAITH

I will call that which allows holding through the suffering in the unfaith, in the empty space, faith. Psychic pain I see as the space where one has surrendered the old, but where one waits experiencing loss and mourning before the spark of new. This capacity to wait initially resides in another, as in the mother and father in the infant's earliest beginnings, or in the therapist in psychoanalytic therapy, or maybe in the patient's memory as a space previously tolerated and chaos previously tolerated to allow the self to reinvent itself. Here, life reoccurs, is born anew, if one can tolerate the psychic pain of surrendering the old and waiting, sustained by faith of the "other." There is a loss of meaning in the daring to surrender what is; there is a tolerating of the terror of possibly falling into nothingness that is an integral part of this. Being in this area of spiritual life is described by the saints as unmitigated, unbearable (yet it must be borne) psychic pain, for in it, the pain of the absence of "God" must needs be tolerated. Only by daring to suffer is the new finding of a new god as an inner psychic reality a possibility.

This chapter is concerned not only with the conditions that allow this space, and the daring to let go to be in it, but with what obstructs the flow of the journey of the psyche to and from it. It is concerned with the timing and dosage, and the relevance of faith as a holding of the dynamic. What in trauma concretizes and forbids or destroys the alive inner space, and what occurs that allows it to become creative, so that one can reinvent oneself? When we say, a person has "lost the faith," we mean there is a deadness, an autistic space where faith would be if it could be, and thinking would be if it could be thought, and feeling could be if we dared to feel.

### The Precreative Space in Taoism

> Since before time and space were,
> The Tao is.
> It is beyond is and is not.
> How do I know this is true?
> I look inside myself and see.
> (Lao-tzu in Stephen Mitchell 1992)

## The Abyss in Judaism

Et tenebrae superfaciem abyssi (Genesis 1:2)—"now the dark was a formless void." The Hebrew word "tehom" translates to abyssus, meaning "depth without ground." The word "abyssus" (from the Greek *abyssos*), "without ground," was a biblical interpolation into Latin. The word occurs forty-two times in the Old Testament.

## In Christianity: Holy Saturday

Friday, Christ died on the cross; Saturday is muted; Sunday, He rose again. Why, in these three days, the supreme drama and central turning point of the Christian religion, is the second day muted, an empty space? "Christ has gone down into the regions of ultimate dread, to the point most distant from God to the darkness that leaves the imagination appalled" (Kelly 1995). The altars lie stripped, the Tabernacles stand empty, and so the muted space for grieving is created. Here then is the black void, and only out of this void can be born the joy of resurrection.

## Mystical Thinking in Early Centuries of the Christian Church

Mystical thinking entailed the idea that the mystic must first have had an experience of union with divine nothingness, which was expressed in the language of the abyss. Saint Augustine in the fourth century defined "abyssus" as "impenetrable and incomprehensible depth, principally applied to a large body of water." Over 900 years later, a mystic of the Middle Ages, John Tauler, was to define it as "the spirit drowned in the bottomless sea" as a result of being part of the eternal spirit of God. Angela of Folingo refers to God as "the abyss, an unknown Nothingness" (*nihil incognitum*). Marguerite Porete, burnt at the stake as a heretic in 1310, wrote: "Now such a soul is nothing. Understanding makes her nothing and places her in nothingness. And so she is all things, from a depth so deep and so great that she finds there neither beginning nor middle nor end, only an abyssal abyss without bottom. There she finds herself without finding and without bottom" (quoted in McGinn 1998, 201)

## Dark Night of the Soul

The darkness is a kind of holy unknowing and is characterized by freedom; it is the opposite of confusion and ignorance. The sense of release in the dark night of the soul is a dying out of desire for the old ways, which become nothing more than habit. The person has by no means forgotten God but remembers God with great pain and grief. Though unable to find Him, the person desires God and is able to forgo particular understanding and comprehension. This is no different from our understanding of the patient who surrenders the old ways of being and struggles in the dark in the paradox, without any hope that will, intellect, or memory can lead anywhere anymore. Saint John and Saint Teresa saw the "purgation" of the night as a healing process in every way. With amazing insight four centuries before Freud, they describe psychological phenomena that would later be called defense mechanisms, behavioral conditioning, addictive disorders, and even psychosis. Mystical thinking was powerfully defensive against sick hallucination, which believed only in its own perverse creations—the mystic believed in the creations of God. Absence actually brings fear and paranoia and, as Bion says, persecution. He shows clearly how an absent space is actually not an absence but the presence of a persecutor. The relevance of an internal object and the holding that internal object gives to the psyche is central to everything I write—as is the waiting in the space for that object to arrive. When one is numbed or frozen, that space cannot be reached.

## AUTISTIC SPACE, DEADNESS, PATHOLOGICAL SPACE

In the precreative space, a psychic event may or may not occur. It holds the pre-conceptive ambivalence of being creative or abortive. What causes our incapacity to open this space and to receive from another? How does the intersection get destroyed after it occurs? How does trauma, undigested or "unsuffered" pain, fear and terror of falling into nothingness, and grasping and incapacity to let go create a situation where the creativity within that space is unable to occur, or where the space is not allowed to open? The traumatized cannot let go; if they do. they fall into the abyss and cannot come out of it. This is an autistic-like space that results from trauma. I am making a very real distinction here between a space where naught "can" occur and a space full of the divine virtues of faith, hope and love, giving meaning—in other words, that things can and will occur. This is an important concept, as it demonstrates the difference between earliest thinking about the evil space that the devil creates, and the ground of the soul, the abyss where the "spark" comes into being from within. Furthermore, in all the work of the saints who speak of this dark night, such as Theresa of Ávila or Thérèse of Lisieux, there is confusion as to whether this is the work of God or of the devil. These spaces are very close together and sometimes hard to differentiate.

## SPACE IN PSYCHOSIS

In psychosis, according to Eigen (2004b, 34), "the very notion of space is in jeopardy. At the other end of the spectrum, the patient's sense of space may be overstuffed and heavy, so that he is unable to resist it." Which therapist among us has not been so incredibly affected by a patient that we feel we have to crawl out of a session and hunch down in the corner of a room trying to recover from a heaviness that consumes the very sense of who we are?

## CASE: VIV

Viv was due to have her baby in three weeks. She has a two-year-old boy. She had been coming to groups off and on for about eight weeks. She was agreeable to having a session with me that we might use for my research on a pregnancy book, so this session was taped. For the first five minutes she sat, not discomfited, just sat. The answers to my questions were not expressive of any emotion. Her eyes were glazed, but there was a hint of sadness in her expression. No emotion was shown at any time during the session. It was not that she did not have any idea what she was doing there, that would be describing an interest in it. During most of the session she sat. They were not awkward spaces. Nothing as alive as that. Finally with some questions from me she began: "The father of my children is not my partner. I live with his mother. He left and I moved in with his mother." It later came out that he had been in remand for "conspiracy to commit a crime." He was not her partner, but he was the father of her children.

"I was in foster care most of my life, probably from when I was about six. My mum is an alcoholic; I don't talk to her anymore. I do have a dad, but he didn't ever live with my mother, it was just an overnight thing. He is also an alcoholic. I lived with my mum again when I was 12 years old. She was still drinking then, and she was pretty violent." I asked, "Was she violent toward you?" She answered, "Yeah, lots! I lived with her for two years from when I was 12 and then I went with my uncle until I was 16, and he looked after me and was good. Both my parents are Aboriginal. I talk to my dad but all he worries about is his drink. At present he's got a choice from the court to dry out or go to jail, so he is trying real hard to dry out. My grandmother on my mother's side was a very strict and stern woman. She never drank. On my father's side my grandmother was so angry no one's ever got really close to her."

I asked, "So was there anyone loving in your life?" "My uncle, my dad's brother, was with my mum a couple of years, and I was with him from when

I was fourteen until I grew up. My uncle, he is like my father, he is the father I never had. I had some illness-mental thing called post-traumatic distress disorder. This was caused by going from one foster home to another. I had nine changes until I was twelve. At twelve I went back to my mother, and she was drinking real heavy like. My uncle was in jail at that time, something to do with driving, and when he got out he went with my mother, but then he left her, and I went with him and he looked after me. My father was jealous. My mother has seven children and my dad has three girls. My brothers and sisters are scattered all over the place."

I asked, "Why did you keep changing foster parents, were you a very difficult child?" "No, I was unhappy. So, they kept moving me on. One family I liked and they were moving to Lismore, and at that point I chose to go home. When things like this happen to you, you learn to just move on, and that is what I spent my life doing, just being unhappy and moving on. I went to year ten in school and when I moved I did a traineeship in administration. I did that for three years. My uncle's still there back home; he's where I go home to. [The company that took me one for the traineeship] do work for the dole and I was an employment consultant. I never had much money. I went there mostly for the experience more than the money. Tom was my first boyfriend, and the first pregnancy was an awful shock I was only eighteen. [The phrase 'awful shock' was repeated four times.] I kind of think of him as my ex-partner. He is in remand. He's been locked up since January and there is still no hearing for a court case. He is really upset that he is missing my son JB and my pregnancy. He was just someone in the wrong place at the wrong time. He is not very happy about it at all. I'm angry because he's not with me, and I don't have any family and he is just not here for me."

I say, "I thought from the first time I saw you, how sad you looked." "Yeah! But I'm here for JB. If it wasn't for JB, I would be on drugs or drink or anything now. He brings me happiness. Tom's mother Tina helps me out with JB. Tom's put me through so much more shit knowing what shit I've been through in my life. Been unhappy for so long I just want to live well and be happy. My [new] baby is a boy. My boys will give me the love I never had. I want to give them a better go than I ever had. JB was nine pounds, eight ounces [just over 4 kilograms]. He is a dynamo and that is why I don't bring him here. He'd tear up the place." She almost comes to life at this point.

Viv was having a baby in three weeks' time and none of the excitement, joy, or interest could be observed, just a strange sad resignation. The only time she lit up and smiled was when I offered to see her through the birth and for the next few months. She did not attend for three sessions, but I kept all her session times open and told her so on the voicemail each time. She spoke to me once and said she was so glad I was there. The abrupt repetitive tearing away in Viv's childhood evoked and recalled and strengthened each prior trauma. Each new home would have been another intruder who transformed her "way of being" by demanding a different existence until there was "no existence" and "you just move on." She deceives us that she is dead, invisible, uninteresting, boring. That is her way of protecting herself from being traumatized again. But it is not true: she is alive and carries life inside her. She is also a "survivor," but what does the identity of "mother" mean for her? A chance to get it right for her children? For them to mother and get it right for her? Both those things? Why, I wondered, are so many young girls getting pregnant as a way of bringing or putting life into the deadness?

I saw Viv with her baby in the hospital. I would love to report how happy she was. Her first remark was "Well, that's over anyway." I got no feeling of joy or response or anything as she held this beautiful baby on her chest. All the comforting trimmings I was used to seeing, of flowers and fruit and chocolates, were totally absent. Her partner had called her from the jail. That was it. I have been seeing her weekly ever since.

## TRAUMA, TRANSGENERATIONAL TRAUMA: THE LEGACY

Maybe it is simplistic to say I see all mental illness as the result of the inability to suffer our suffering. The dose has been too large, or the timing all wrong, the infant asked to carry too much. The protective cover of our being is ripped, and we spill out or, worse, shatter into a thousand pieces. There are fathers and mothers who cannot suffer their own suffering. They powerfully, unconsciously, have the children suffer it for them. We see children all the time who suffer the pain of the previous generations. Two examples come most markedly to my mind: children of the survivors of the Holocaust, and Muslim children, of immigrant parents, who choose to blow themselves to smithereens rather than tolerate the suffering their parents tolerated. Also, there are the dire results of the generational suffering of Aboriginal people visited on the present Aboriginal people in a way that sometimes makes them quite criminal, as if paying us back now for what others did to their parents not so long ago. Old women on the block buy drugs from Lebanese gangs to give to their own kids. Ironically, the children of the dispossessed sell to the dispossessed. All we hold sacred in motherhood and culture is being challenged here.

Michael Eigen's writing has been so influential in all that I write here. See his chapters on "The Core of Psychosis" and "Mindlessness" in *The Psychotic Core* (2004b), as well as *The Electrified Tightrope* (1993) and *Psychic Deadness* (2004a). Eigen penned this piece in our online discussion:

> At the core of psychotic states is trauma. The core of trauma is disaster. A disaster has befallen the personality. Whether it is a chemical disaster, an inherited disaster, a physiological disaster, an environmental disaster, something awful has happened to oneself, to one's personality, to growth and development. Something is off, something catastrophic has happened, and one doesn't know what to do with it. One is stuck with it, and it feels hopeless. Here we are dealing with a powerful anti-life force. This force that goes on destroying after it destroys everything. You get destruction swallowing lust for life, absorbing it, destroying it. This destruction is darker, bleaker, deadlier—not a lustful war, but a "lustless" one that has its own momentum, its own force, gradient, vector. The deadness Bion is pointing to is the failure of the birth and growth of animism or aliveness. The deadness Bion is attempting to communicate is beyond the something more deadly. If any libido or pleasure comes near it, it is swallowed up, destroyed, blackholed. All it needs is its own deadly deadness, i.e., nothing, in this case the deadliest nothing beyond imagining. But it will not be the deadness that makes animism impossible, that deadens, forecloses, ends all animism, that makes it impossible for animism to begin. I think it is important to stare into the heart of this deadness because it exerts a momentous force on all other deaths which are amalgamated with pleasure and dreams, waking or sleeping. (Mike Eigen, from a personal correspondence, May 2006)

Trauma turns living space into a non-living, non-thinking, autistic-like space; a sterile womb that deadens all that enters it—nothing can live in it. This is a powerful antilife force, a self-destructiveness that may be born in the person created by generations of not being or not feeling wanted. For Aboriginal people, this is not a feeling that is from the past, but is alive right now in the present, deeply entrenched and active in their psyche. They have not only adopted the hatred of the other but have integrated it as self-hatred. It is like a dark vortex where everything that is alive, or even has the potential to live, is drawn in the vortex, sucked into itself and destroyed. This negative force is inculcated through generations until it is digested and becomes part of being. It is not limited to Aboriginal people; it is present in many, maybe most, maybe all of us. No birth can occur if that deadly power is greater than the living one. The paradigm is of an awful mother continuously aborting an infant in her womb. So deep and total is the destructiveness, that abortion is of our sensory pleasure, of all desire, of all living experience. The sucking in to destroy in trauma results in deadened autistic space. The problem of psychosis is that it has perverted and stultified chaos rather than making its way through it. Why do we incorporate the self our parents see us as, and how the world we live in views us? Why does this so potently live with us through our lives? How does this stuff enter us? If we knew this, we might know how to help Aboriginal mothers not feel like they are "a piece of shit," which is the exact term they use about themselves. How did the Aboriginal people over thousands of eons deal with their trauma? Here, they tell us, is their greatest gift to us—the gift of Dadirri.

## Dadirri

These reflections are taken from "Dadirri: Listening to one another," by Daly River Aboriginal artist, Miriam-Rose Ungunmerr:

> Dadirri is about tapping into the dead springs within us. Aboriginal people have a special respect for nature. The identity we have with the land is sacred and unique. We also have a strong sense of community. All persons matter—all of us belong. In our language it is called Dadirri, where we share and reach into our deep spring. It is inner, deep listening and quiet, still "awareness." A big part of Dadirri is listening. Throughout the years, we have sat in circles and we have listened to our stories. In the circle the one in pain speaks, the others listen. We own that grief, we share that grief and this allows it to heal slowly. In Dadirri, the circle, a person is in pain or trouble, he speaks out to his pain and trouble. We sit in a circle around the person. We have his pain, this heals it. This is Dadirri. (Ungunmerr 2003, vii–ix)

> In Dadirri spirit, the spirit of God is a sound, it is the sound of God calling, of deep calling. It is the spirit of Dadirri, it is the place before we were born, before we were in our mother's womb. So, we let him touch this deep pain place and begin to heal. (Ungunmerr 2003, vii–ix)

> Through the years we have listened to the stories. In our aboriginal way, we learn to listen from our earliest days. We could not live good and useful lives unless we listen. This was the normal way for us to learn—not by asking questions. We learnt by watching and listening, waiting and then acting. Our people have passed on this way of listening for over 40,000 years. (Ungunmerr 2003, vii–ix)

## Violence

> The wilful denigration and destruction of Aboriginal ceremonial responsibilities and processes by the colonizers has therefore had profound transgenerational effects on the people of this land. Aboriginal people have been prevented from engaging in ceremonial processes for healing from the trauma. The distressed feelings that accompany loss, death and devastation remain as destructive forces within the land and the people. (Atkinson 2002, 35)

> The psychological impact of the experiences of dispossession, degeneration and degradation are beyond description. They strike at the very core of a sense of being and identity . . . anger, despair, abusiveness. The effects are generational . . . I realised that it was a miracle that we weren't all stark, raving mad. (O'Shane 1995, 151–53)

## CASE: LOREENA

I want to use this case to discuss the impact of the loss of her baby on an eighteen-year-old Aboriginal mother, as well as her journey through a subsequent birth and a further pregnancy. The period she is in therapy is the first eighteen months of her second infant's life and the pregnancy and birth of her third baby. I hope to show how the intergenerational nature of trauma in her own family of origin, her own mother's surrender of her in her infancy, the environment of violence and addiction in which she grew up, impacted her response to the loss of her infant, and affected her journey through adolescence and her journey as mother to her new babies. Loreena had had an abortion at fifteen years of age, a pregnancy terminating in the stillbirth of a girl baby at sixteen years of age, and a further pregnancy and a healthy baby boy by the time therapy began. The account here is partly written by an Aboriginal health worker who saw Loreena on a mostly weekly basis; I was the supervisor and we called in for discussion a child psychoanalytic therapist based in London, whose special area of concern is infant death and its effect on future pregnancies. This degree of support made possible a degree of mourning and consequent growth that otherwise would have been very difficult, if not impossible—but it was not enough.

### Cultural Background Thinking

Urban Aboriginal women face quite distinct challenges relating to pregnancy and bringing up young infants. Many of the women we see who have lost babies in this generation, had mothers or grandmothers who were part of the "stolen generation." Aboriginal mothers have been dislocated in time, dislocated from their land, dislocated from their culture, their community and their own families. The failure to resolve this dislocation, as with any trauma, leads to symptoms of violence or drug and alcohol abuse, and this was certainly the case for the settlement where Loreena grew up in Victoria, Australia. In her violence was the enactment of the violence she experienced through the loss of her own mother who gave her away in infancy, the lies and deceit around this, the death of her first infant, and finally a sense of hopeless loss in her community. "We are a dead people," she said once, "there is no hope for us.

You look into our eyes, and you see dead people. We are finished. We are all of us dead!" She tried to solve her personal sense of violation by violating herself through drugs and alcohol in early adolescence and was saved by the school counselor; ever since that positive experience, she always found someone who would "save" or protect her.

## Loreena's History

Loreena's mother had given her up in early infancy or perhaps even from birth. The paranoia and sense of powerlessness that we saw in Loreena was typical of the Aboriginal women we work with. Her violent breakouts that we saw in severe crisis times were a response to that sense of helplessness, and the lack of power to affect or change her environment. This sense of loss pervaded her community. Loreena was raised mostly by her "Nana" (not her biological grandmother) who lived in Queensland in an Aboriginal settlement. When Loreena was a baby, her biological mother abandoned her to the woman whom Loreena thought of as her mother until one day, when she was thirteen years old, Loreena came home from school and found everyone sniggering as she walked in. They started to tease her, "Who do you think your mother is?" Loreena was totally shocked to discover that a woman who lived down the road, who she knew and whose children she knew, was her real mother. The women all thought it was a big joke. Loreena did not see the funny side. She became suicidal and delinquent, hating both her foster mother and her own mother. When at fifteen she became pregnant, she had an abortion because she hated the boy she was with; she now says she does not regret the abortion. Loreena then ran away to Sydney. She was picked up by DOCS (Child Care Services) and placed with a twenty-four-year-old Koori woman as a foster mother. Realizing that she was heading down the wrong path with the alcohol and drugs, Loreena took herself back to school and got her HSC, but in the final year at school she became pregnant by John. This baby, Tiuana, was stillborn, and John, who was only seventeen at this time, left Loreena and went off with another girl. Months later John returned, and Loreena quickly became pregnant again with Jimmy, and six weeks after this live birth she became pregnant again. Here is part of the first session as recorded by her therapist, a young Aboriginal worker who I had supervised for many years:

> When I came in I could see she had been crying. She apologized and explained that she and her partner John, the father of the two babies, Tiuana (stillborn) and Jimmy, a beautiful little boy who is now six weeks old, had been quarreling a lot lately. She hated him, she said. When Tiuana was born they separated. They got together for Tiuana's funeral, but after the funeral they separated again. Loreena

then didn't see John for five months; she was angry because she didn't think that John had grieved for their girl and he seemed unable to understand how she felt: "I am not my normal happy self." Loreena explained that she had started to feel sick and she couldn't feel Tiuana moving. She told John that she needed to go to the doctor. Then she had the ultrasound, and sadly she learned that the baby was dead. She was taken into hospital, where the doctor explained what he needed to do to get Tiuana out. Loreena said the nurses and doctors let her stay with Tiuana and hold her all that day. They took photos of Tiuana, which Loreena keeps in a shoebox. She got the shoebox out to show me. It was decorated with pink paper and ribbon. It was very sad, as here was a baby who had been dead in the womb for at least four weeks. They gave her some medication, which made her feel as if she was detached from herself—she couldn't remember much after that. Loreena paid attention to Jimmy through all this talking. The baby was in the bouncinette and every so often Loreena would pick him up and cuddle him. Loreena said that she sometimes imagined Jimmy with Tiuana's face. This, she said, helped her to cope. Loreena blames herself for Tiuana's death. She said that she took vitamins right through her pregnancy. She said the hospital had told her that the cause of Tiuana's death was the wall of the uterus giving way. [Excerpt from case notes]

Loreena showed no emotion in this first interview and there was a deadened quality to her narration, even though she said so much. The worker felt extremely worried for Loreena. We were aware of the degree of ambivalence and confusion around the various issues, such as who is this living baby? Where does the blame lie for the other baby's death? Hatred and love for the partner were so confused. Fragmentation brought on by birth had the added stress of unresolved grief. One day Loreena sent her worker a text message asking her to phone as soon as she could. She sounded upset and explained that she had run amok the night before, lost control, trashed the house, broke the windows, and gone crazy. A friend of Loreena's talked about John and his relationship with another girl. When John came home, Loreena was angry with him and started to question him about that relationship. That was when she trashed the house and attacked John with a knife. She said that she cut John's arm before he managed to grab her and hold her down until he was too tired to fight anymore. Loreena rang the worker again the next day, and a kind of terrifying chase for her occurred along the train stations. Finally, she told the worker she was with her mother-in-law. There was a new kind of depression as she told the worker that when she was fourteen she had gone off the rails. She started drinking, smoking, and experimenting with drugs; she also attempted suicide. "I don't want to go there again," she said. Here is some of what the health worker wrote:

> Loreena started to cry. She felt hurt because she couldn't understand how her real mother could look after her sometimes and never tell her that she was her mother, and also spend time with the other children and not have time to raise Loreena and love her. Loreena said she couldn't talk about her feelings in a way that anyone understood, and that this was why she had become mentally unbalanced. (Excerpt from case notes)

This inability to give words, and therefore access, to their feelings is a common problem for Aboriginal women. In part, this powerlessness on Loreena's part is the result of the trauma of the loss of her baby, and this "not being heard" comes from very far back in her history: "I am haunted by the images of the mothers screaming and howling with grief as 'the welfare' took their children from them. The 'white man' with the infants and children in the trucks did not, would not, hear their cries."

When not heard one becomes numb. Our supporting supervisor from the Tavistock Clinic in London wrote, "I like your idea that there is a sense of an inner space that becomes deadened and cut off. Do you think with women who have lost babies that this space represents the uterus, and that there is a phantasy that takes a rather concrete form that the uterus contributed in some way to the death? This becomes a death-dealing space rather than a nurturing one, the black hole in the mind becomes the black hole of the uterus. When a baby dies the good internal mother dies also, and she is left at the mercy of internal, persecutory, destructive mother forces." The supervisor wondered whether, when a mother loses a baby, the mother also feels she has lost a part of herself. This in turn leads to a real feeling that a part of the self is gone and can never be replaced. She wrote, "I thought about fear of loss, fear of losing her partner and I thought: 'How, with this cultural history, can there be any sense of stability?' A fear of being attached, falling in love. Her identity, such as it was, appears to have been shot to pieces by both the loss and the birth." The health worker wrote:

> Loreena talked for the first time about Tiuana's birth. It was a natural birth and she was in labor for ten hours. She was on pethidine and off the planet. She asked John, "Why am I here?" and John cried and said, "You are going to give birth to a little baby girl, but she is dead." Loreena remembered the nurses taking photos of Tiuana and how she felt angry and upset about this. I asked her, "What about the night nurse? You were angry with her, weren't you?" She became visibly upset, although she was not crying, and said, "The night nurse tried to take Tiuana off me, saying, 'Enough is enough! You have to let go of her now.'" Loreena tried to ring John to try to stop her from taking Tiuana from her. He and her foster mother came to the hospital to be with her. "I wasn't ready to let Tiuana go," she said. "At that point I died." (Excerpt from case notes)

After the birth of her second baby Loreena went beserk again. This time she did not wreck the house. This time she called the therapist. There were six messages in all over the period from midnight to 3 in the morning. In the messages Loreena spoke of how desperate she was, and how she felt John did not love her and was only with her because of the babies. The health worker went to Loreena first thing next morning. Loreena talked a lot with the worker about the new baby but was very sad for quite some time, as if she was again in mourning. The worker was aware of how, instead of running away on the train, Loreena was still at home and very caring and skilled in the way she handled her baby. Possum, the baby, was still curling up a little bit; he actually looked at her now, not quite smiling, but a beautiful baby. "He is a bit restless at the moment," Loreena said, "but it could be because of how I'm feeling." She now, instead of enacting her anger, could experience it and call for help.

Aboriginal young men are infamous for leaving their partners and moving away from them to other women. We felt proud of the worker for being able to help Loreena to hold on to John, albeit with some pain and difficulty. Loreena was now beginning to talk about looking for work. She had a fear of being housebound with two small children. She was even thinking of asking John's mother to mind them while she went out to work.

I wish I could report on how we did good work with this one case, but I am not at all sure I can. Loreena started working in an institution for two days a week. The staff had one of their many parties there, and Loreena stayed and got very drunk. She was seduced by an older female member of staff. She could not stop damaging herself and used it against herself, revealing it in an interview with her partner's work counselor. Her partner took the children and left, going back to his parents. Loreena overdosed, but she did call our worker. The worker could hear that her voice was slurred and called the police. What happened next was the worker who had visited Loreena dozens of times could not remember the name of her street. She phoned the previous worker who also could not remember it. The worker finally did find it through a Google Earth search, so the police could locate her. Loreena ran away soon after leaving her babies. She has returned and is keeping in touch with them, and despite drinking a great deal has managed a job from time to time. All we hoped for in the breaking of transgenerational trauma seemed to have failed. Loreena did just what her mother did to her. The anger and the helplessness remain, and so does the despair for any of us doing this work. But there is the possibility of hope.

> The quotation here is an Aboriginal man's telling of the day his baby was born and seeing him for the first time:
> In its own Wunder place

A spirit waits for birth
today, I saw him the child he really is
That is how a man learns to know his child.
(Isaacs 2005)

## ACKNOWLEDGMENTS

I want to acknowledge the help and support of Jeff Eaton, who contributed to the first part of this chapter in daily conversation with me. Jeff is part of the song line, the dreaming that extended from subterranean Sydney to subterranean New York with the Mike Eigen online discussion group and on to Seattle, where Jeff lives and works. I acknowledge as always the work of Mike as a generous friend and mentor to Jeff and myself.

Chryne Griffiths was the Aboriginal worker who stayed with Loreena through all this time. Marguerite Reid from the Chelsea and Westminster Hospital, London deserves our gratitude for supervising my supervision of Loreena's case for two full years by email.

Quoted with kind permission from the publisher Trauma Trails, *Recreating Song Lines: The Transgenerational Effects of Trauma in Indigenous Australia*, Judy Atkinson, Spinifex Press, 2002.

Precreative Space, Norma Tracey The Psychoanalytic Review Volume 96, Issue 6 December 2009. Reprinted with permission of Guilford Press.

# *Chapter 11*

# Working With Traumatized Aboriginal Infants and Children in Early Years of Life

> Please don't let the crocodile eat me. (Three-year-old Aboriginal child)

> Indigenous people are the most disadvantaged group within Australia across the full spectrum of socio-economic indicators. (*National Indigenous English Literacy and Numeracy Strategy 2000–2004*)

Aboriginal people are the most important people to the Aboriginal nation. They are the carers, the healers that give emotional empowerment to their children. As partners, not claiming possession, not politicking care for small children, the hope is that we professionals, Aboriginal and non-Aboriginal, can work together to create the one opportunity to neutralize and heal the trauma that so many Aboriginal infants and small children experience in their early years. This is the one chance from pregnancy and early childhood years to bring the best of our experiences and learning to help their mothers and fathers to be supported in their care.

The responsiveness of the psyche at this tender age allows growth in a way that may never again be available during life. This chapter addresses not only traumatized children, but traumatized mothers and fathers, sometimes a transgenerational traumatized community, where past and present experiences have combined to create the unbearable suffering of trauma. The chapter combines Aboriginal cultural Dreamtime concepts with psychoanalytic thinking and over sixty years' experience of working with pregnant women, mothers and infants and mothers of young children.

What is the nature of infant and early childhood trauma? How do we counter this in our practice and in our centers? What specific techniques act as guidelines in our daily task of working with traumatized children, as we move from trauma and its healing, from theory to pragmatic reality in what we do? How can we improve our skills in this area? What new initiatives can we attempt? What are the specific needs of our Aboriginal children? How do we share more of our cultural knowledge and the creation stories of the Dreamtime in a way that make our children proud to be Aboriginal? Creating our own CDs of song and dance; producing booklets for parents; allowing creative play inclusive of myths, culture and tradition; growing bush tucker and veggie gardens; using dancing, drama and art as forms of healing; improving pre-literacy programs are just some of the practical ways.

But first there is a question of who cares for the teachers, while the teachers care for the child. How does one work when the work touches the core of one's own traumas? For the staff, trauma workshops, debriefing, drama enactments, and supportive supervision must be integral parts of their work, so they can create a holistic program best suited to these traumatized children? How can parents be helped so that they are not afraid to extend their learning, so that they can improve their understanding of what their children are learning, and support and give praise for what they have achieved?

How successful are government programs such as Families First and Brighter Futures? How do we access these to support our work, forming partnerships rather than rivalry and suspicion?

Are many Aboriginal children traumatized? Are their parents traumatized? Are the Aboriginal staff at the centers traumatized? How one grows out of trauma and understands its impediment to growth is of the utmost relevance.

## PSYCHIC SPACE

The idea of psychic space speaks to a place in the mind for receiving, listening and creating; it is about a space for emotional growth. In this space, a person creates the meaning of our world from out of their own thinking. In this space the world is imagined into being. Aboriginal people have been doing this for centuries. In the Dreamtime were the creation stories.

It is a recreating of our world from our imagining. "How do we dream? Who is the dreamer that we do not, cannot ever know, who does our dreaming?" (Grotstein 2000, 357). Who makes up and imbues meaning into the world around us? Ancient Aboriginals talked of "singing yourself into existence"; this is known as autochthony. Some internal self, unknown and unknowable to the conscious self, is active always in the unconscious, working all the time to make up and dream self, and dream those around self into existence, and so creating one's own myths. This is in tension always with the idea of the other, and how others see the person, philosophically known as alterity. This continual creating of self, of others in our world and of the environs we live in, is our Aboriginal dreaming that goes on and on. "You can kill people, but nothing can kill the dreaming" (Barry Smith, personal communication to author, 2005).

## The Interrelatedness of All Living Things: Giving Meaning to the World Around Us

This place to create a place to be is at the very basis of all psychic being. Trauma kills this space; trauma destroys the capacity to fantasize; trauma kills dreaming. Preschool and early school work with free play, stories, song and dance, art, growing things, crafting, recreating this dreaming space. It creates space and allows children to create the world as they want to, rather than through harsh imposition from without by trauma. The preschool center is the concept of the sacred sites, a sacred, safe, secure space where trauma heals. That space gives holding, reliability, security, learning to handle stimulus that is appropriate in timing and dose, and allows the possibility of life—a precreative space to be.

## What Happens in Trauma for the Infant, the Small Child?

Trauma creates a stimulus beyond what the little child can cope with—the terror of death at the core of all traumas. Trauma loses the holding of an alive mother in the mind. Trauma destroys the holding womb of the mind. Trauma destroys the core self. Trauma creates a numbness, an autistic space, a void. Trauma kills the space in the psyche to create. Trauma kills dreaming. It is like a vortex that sucks in and kills all life. The earlier the event, or continuing events, the more they affect the child for the rest of his or her life.

## Trauma Blocks out the Creative Space: Trauma Kills Dreaming

At the center of all trauma is violent emotion, beyond the child's capacity to suffer. The internal holding womb collapses and becomes a sterile womb that deadens all emotion. Central is a deadened and deadening internal mother. The good mother's internalized containing womb is shattered. That which holds that core self, part that is unknown and unknowable, is violated. Trauma ruptures this central core self in a way that is horrifying to conceive. It aborts the fetal self. The central core becomes a "no person." The living womb space becomes a non-living, non-thinking, autistic-like space. Sensitive sense of self is fragmented, negative fears are greater than positive hopes. There is no creative space. The inner world becomes a dark, frightening abyss instead of a safe and protective place. Life is rooted in abject fear and terror, freezing all emotion and joy in living. Sometimes bits of emotion break through—nightmares. The child no longer has the potential to dream or sing itself into existence. The child grasps reality as a defense against dreaming; grasps acquisitions because the capacity to dream is dead.

This is passed on to the next generation, with terrible consequences. It is passed on because the mother, not having her core self, cannot hold the child in a way that sustains the child's core self (LaMothe 2012, 870). Babies have no meaning if the psychic mother is dead; our children lose their sacred meaning—what is left is hopelessness, depression, lack of self-esteem, feeling of worthlessness, drugs, drinking, suicide. No dreaming left! A living nightmare! The dead do not dream.

The family, the Aboriginal mob, and the preschool center can be places of trauma or a healing space, a living womb in which the child can grow. This can be the psychic space of the dreaming or the place of nightmares. It can be a preschool space where the small child can fantasize, symbolize, and create through free play, creative arts, tending gardens, and just being. In this safe neutral space, children can learn; they can be free to think without fearing the thoughts will become real, they can have a space to experiment and test out. This shows the relevance of the creative space for healing the traumatized child.

### What Heals Trauma?

A safe space to be at home, at preschool; a safe place to fantasize, to play, to express through art, dance, song, mime, puppets, building and creating; a space that is secure and predictable. A good enough parent can initially create this space for the infant and small child, but a good enough child center creates it in countless important ways. The child center is a safe place where through therapy the workers can neutralize what has been traumatic for the child, the emotions that have been too much for them in their young and sensitive life.

## CASE: ADAM

Adam's father is Aboriginal, he is a former boxer and according to the mother, "had one too many punches to the head." She also tells me that Adam, far from being planned, was conceived "between glasses of beer." She said it was just her luck to get pregnant to such a loser. At the birth the father was high on Rohies (Rohypnol) and so disruptive, that the Department of Community Services (DoCS) at first refused to allow her to take the infant home. Although she had left three previous children with her first husband, she fought very hard to keep this one.

Adam is a three-and-a-half-year-old Aboriginal. He attends an inner city childcare center three days a week. I worked as a consultant to that center. This is a narrative of how we at the center worked to encourage this little boy to move his journey from the world of "acting out" into the world of inner fantasy, and how he learned to enact the dreaming and the terrible fears and challenges of his life through play.

As a teenager, Adam's mother, Gemina got in with a "bad crowd," went on drugs, and is now on methadone. She is extremely thin and gaunt, and she looks undernourished. She has had a series of "unsuitable" partners, and Adam's father was in jail for a year for assault and robbery. The director and staff originally brought Adam to my attention because they were seriously concerned by his behavior. His mother had recently taken a partner, to whom Adam was attached. But one Monday morning, Adam told the staff that this partner had stabbed his mother in the leg the previous Saturday night. Gemina was taken to hospital. It is possible that both were drunk, and there were reports from the neighbors and police of mutual violence.

Although Adam was fully toilet trained, he was now wetting himself, even defecating in a bucket instead of the toilet, attacking other children, and being erratic and aggressive. One morning a father had come to the center with his son. Adam ran round and round in uncontained circles, madly throwing toys everywhere, and attacked and punched the father even though he was known to him. He was so out of control the director held him physically and took him into another room to settle him. All the staff spoke about him in the discussion, agreeing that he acted like a real toughie, like a teenage street kid.

I referred Adam for special work with the childcare worker and I supervised every session. In the worker's first session with Adam, she explained that he would have special playtime with her, that she had special toys he could play with during these times. He seemed to understand immediately, was most responsive, and eagerly chose to play with the felt bears out of the box. They were figures from the story of the three bears. The worker reported what happened next:

> Adam manipulated all the felt pieces quickly, becoming engrossed in his play. He showed really strong emotions towards mummy bear. She was kissed and cuddled and he rubbed her leg. "Mummy bear's got a sore leg," he said, "I'll take her to the doctor." He then picked up daddy bear and said, "I will punch you, big bear," and proceeded to. I asked, "Why are you punching father bear?" Adam said, "He is naughty! Very naughty! I will throw him outside." He stood up, opened the window of the playhouse, and threw him out. He was very angry. He then came back and looked at the mummy bear, and said, "If you're naughty

> you'll go outside too." He then cuddled mummy bear, cuddled baby bear, and then threw mummy bear out the window. I asked, "Why is mummy bear outside?" He replied, "She is naughty too! She's very naughty, so she goes outside too.' He waited a while and then talked to both of them. "If you are sorry and you say sorry, you can come back in, but if you're naughty you go out again." He then brought them both in and placed them on the cushion in the playhouse. (Excerpt from her case notes)

In discussion, we thought in his fantasy that Adam is courageous enough to beat up on the big bear, but in reality he must be terrified of his lack of power and of his incapacity to manage violence. In fantasy he is in control, so he can create punishment for father and mother bear's naughtiness. The trauma is that the events are not controllable. Once he can get control and throw the naughty emotions out, he can forgive mummy and daddy bear and bring them back inside his inner world. He warns them, however, that if they become naughty, that is, if the negative emotions overwhelm him, he will have no choice but to punish them by putting them outside his mind.

Adam became a great worry to the staff at many points. One was when he pursued little girls into a hiding place and asked them to take off their pants as he had an erection. He did this with his special worker too. We called in a child psychiatrist who told us that little children did have sex play. Not like this they didn't, and Adam would often comment to the worker who gave him his afternoon nap, "I am a big man now, I can do sex."

Over the year, Adam's play became extremely rich and varied. Suddenly in one of the sessions a make-believe baby appeared. For weeks he threw it in the garbage, as it was "no good." Then one day he told his worker, "I might just let this baby lie between us." Then he started taking on aspects of a baby. Adam started to ask if he could play in the babies' room. Each time the ritual was that they would go to the babies' room and ask the head teacher for permission to enter and play. One day he lay on the floor and sucked at a baby's bottle. He said to his worker, "You didn't know that baby was me, did you?" All the staff became aware of how vulnerable he had become. He would often cry and ask for a cuddle. This change came after a lot of play with a teddy, and later with a doll that the worker brought for him. For days at the center he sat protecting the sleeping doll, and telling the others to be very quiet and not disturb the baby. His sex play disappeared. He showed himself a leader, often telling others what was, and what was not, OK to do. Where once he used to grab his food like a little animal, now he became particularly adept with his handling of his meals and could wait for his turn. He loved stories and group play but would wait and put his hand up to answer a question. The saddest part is that his mother seems to have no awareness of his vulnerability. He works and works to invite her interest in his play, and so do the staff. She is still on methadone, and drinks to the point of arriving tipsy to pick him up.

The enormous thing Adam has learned over the year of therapy is how to fantasy in his play instead of act in his life. So, what is the miracle that transforms? Hearing, listening, allowing the stories to be told. Pain shared is pain diminished. Crying is a sign of hope, a sign of still fighting for life. A teacher said, "It is the children who cannot cry that we worry about. They may be no trouble but you're aware that the joy of living is gone from them."

## EMOTIONAL LISTENING: DADIRRI

Ancient Aboriginal culture knew about trauma and its healing, as I have discussed in earlier Chapters. Dadirri and the ideas of the Dreaming and the role of listening from the depth of our souls was well known to Aboriginal people.

## CASE: ALANA

A young Aboriginal couple sit with me in my clinic room. Their three-year-old plays happily on the floor with a teddy. She has a shawl she wraps teddy in, putting him to sleep and tending most caringly to him. She seems oblivious of the doors that have opened to pain in both her parents, I think. She is in a bubble, safe from it, but then I think she *is* the sleeping teddy protected from the pain. A palpable blackness fills the room. I cannot avoid it. I am in it. I feel and see and smell it. I wish I was anywhere but in that space.

Her mother Jeno looks at me and cries, "When I have to beg for a hug from Tom, I feel degraded. I feel like a piece of sh . . . , like I am a nothing and no one, and still he can't see or hear me." She sobs. "All my life I have felt like a piece of useless sh. . ., and he just makes sure that I keep feeling that way. He reminds me every day I am worthless, a no one."

Pain meets pain. But the silence is deadly, and I am sure he is not speaking because he has no words. It is a relief when after five minutes he finds some: "So do you think I was born with a silver spoon in my mouth or somethin'? There weren't no father around, just my mother. I had to take care of myself, there wasn't anyone else. I work for you like a bloody dog, but it is never enough, never good enough. Sometimes I get home and you are on the computer, and I feel I just want to break that bloody computer to pieces. There is bloody dog shit everywhere, no room for me, your bloody dogs are more important than I am. On the $4000 lounger there is dog shit, can't get to the toilet to do a piss without walking in dog shit! I feel like kicking the buggers out. No room for me—the dogs have all the room!"

He is the dog shit. The beautiful child plays on the floor, awakens teddy, plays with him a little then wraps teddy up and puts him to bed again, talking gently and comfortingly to him.

I feel palpably their anger, hurt, rage, and blackness as they leave me. How much pain can any human being suffer? They look accusingly at me for exposing and witnessing their suffering, but they are grateful someone has heard it.

## CAN TRAUMA BE INHERITED?

There is now adequate evidence that trauma can affect the DNA and be transmitted to the next generation. This is frightening knowledge and makes the work we do with the children of this generation even more serious.

### Pregnancy

For Aboriginal women, pregnancy and birth were among the most sacred of events. The land where the birth took place was sacred. It remained sacred for the whole of that child's life. This has been fractured. A sacred place of birth is lost, right in their own bodies. Our Aboriginal women need to know from the moment of conception that smoking, drug and alcohol abuse, domestic violence, and high emotional stress all interfere seriously with the cortisol growth hormones of their unborn infant. We now know that in the womb an infant's cortisol levels can be interfered with by one event of domestic violence or by more than a month of drug taking.

### Affect Regulation and Early Years

The first three years of a child's life are more critical to their lifelong development and chances than previously recognized. Nurturing and supportive relationships established from birth positively affect brain development and, equally, stress (as experienced in domestic violence situations) and lack of bonding and attachment to parents and caregivers can adversely affect babies' brain development. These experiences can affect the neurons in the brain that are responsible for learning and emotional development and have a lifetime impact (Fish 2002 as cited by Flood 2006).

A diverse group of disciplines have intensified their attention upon the scientific study of emotion. Studies of the human infant brain demonstrate that its maturation is influenced by the environment and is dependent on experience. It is particularly dependent on the mother's early capacity to create and help with affect regulation—affect means emotional state, and regulation means control. Mothers teach their children how to self-regulate.

From in the womb, neuron pathways are laid down in response to our environment—a thousand million changes a second, as our bodies adapt to the environment. Millions of interactive messages create responses within the fetus, infant and child, adolescent, adult for the whole of their lives, but the main ones are set in the first four years of life. For example, studies have shown that infants not exposed to socialization will have smaller social areas of the brain than infants exposed to socialization within the first six months of life. Schore (1998) says the relationship between early failures of development and a predisposition to later development of emotional disturbance is a central issue for all childcare workers.

## PSYCHOBIOLOGICAL BASIS

As I noted in Chapter 6, research now compels us to view ourselves as an integrated physiological and psychological unit. There is no question that the effects of trauma in infancy shows how the psychological results of trauma have biological antecedents, and this has been the basis of all our work as therapists; emotional neglect in infancy can cause major changes in the pathways of emotional response.

Trauma, whether singular or accumulated, can create areas or pockets of autism, can be dissociated and repressed, and then reawakened through the psychophysical events of pregnancy and birth, and in this way are also passed on to the next generation. Using an interdisciplinary approach, researchers such as Schore, who wrote *Affect Regulation and the Origin of the Self* (1994), have shown that social factors modulate the biological structure of the brain. The brain's self-organizing occurs in the context of a relationship with another "self" or another brain. Studies have shown that a child's IQ level can be reduced by as much as 40 percent by social situations and showed that stimulus given to different areas of the brain at crucial sensitive stages considerably affects growth.

### Attachment

Infant work from all disciplines offers knowledge of an attachment bond of affective communication. The failure of the dyad to create this bond is central to the transmission of emotional disorders across generations. It is well known that the emotions that flow between mother and child, every moment that they share and negotiate together, affects the infant and its inner psyche emotionally and physically. Every experience shapes the organization of a regulatory system in the orbital frontal-limbic areas of the right hemisphere.

It is an important concept that can bridge the "mind–body" gap. The essential task of the first year of human life is the creation of a secure attachment bond between the infant and the primary caregiver. Attachment is built into the nervous system. The brain literally requires brain interaction that occurs in the context of a positive affective relationship between mother and infant (Trevarthen 1998, 63).

## Attunement

The more a mother tunes her activity level to the infant during periods of social engagement, the more she allows her child to recover quietly in periods of disengagement, and the more she contingently responds to signals for reengagement, the more synchronised their interaction. Mutually attuned interactions are fundamental to the ongoing affective development of the infant. In light of the fact that mis-attunement often happens normally, the mother must modulate non-optimal high levels of stimulation that would induce super-high levels of arousal in the infant, and, most importantly, must participate in interactive repair to regulate stressful infant states. Psychobiological attunement is the fundamental mechanism that mediates attachment bond formation (Field, Diego and Hernandez-Reif 2010).

The emotional experiences of the young child develop through sounds, images and pictures, and these are stored or processed in the brain's right hemisphere during the formative stages. The hard wiring of circuits in the child's right cortex will come to mediate his thinking feeling capacities. This right hemisphere is dominant in human infants in the first four years of life. Neurobiological studies show that the orbital frontal cortex, which is enlarged in the right hemisphere, acts as the highest level of control of behavior, especially in relation to emotion. Early deprivation of empathic care, either in the form of excessive arousal reduction or intensification, creates a growth-inhibiting environment.

Disorders of attachment we now know beyond doubt are at the core of psychopathology. These early failures of self-regulation and interactional attunement lie at the very basis of all future social and personal problems. What a heavy message. These failures create a limited capacity to moderate or handle the intensity and the length of the affect. All forms of psychopathology have, in part, symptoms of emotional dysregulation, mainly as a result of growth inhibition. Loss of ability to regulate the intensity of feelings is the most far-reaching effect of early trauma and neglect.

### Negotiated Moments: Attunement, Jeremiah and The Crocodile

We now know that the life a child has with its mother in the beginning and onwards for the whole of its life is made up of negotiated moments. This is an example from a preschool:

> The teacher sits on the floor, legs spread slightly, as Jeremiah, who has a slight intellectual disability, puts large wooden pieces together on the floor, with careful non-intrusive help. She asks what it is he is making. "It is my boat," he says with a degree of pride. "Oh, I will get on the boat," says Nathan, and jumps on. Jeremiah angrily pushes Nathan over. "He got on my boat!" he cries. The teacher goes to the children and holds them both. "Jeremiah, remember the rule, we never push—we share! You have such a nice boat, Nathan wanted to share it with you. Why don't the three of us sing a song about sharing and then maybe you can both get on the boat." As they clap, hold hands, and sing, some of the others wander over and join in the song. Jeremiah is gifted with music and singing. The teacher tells me that because Jeremiah is a really big boy, he has to be taught that he can use his strength for good things, or he may end up not accepted at any school or by any kids. "He has no awareness of how to use his strength, but he is much improved, and we try to give him one-on-one time each day. We are going to keep him here another year, so that he will be more ready for school in an intellectual and social sense."

Talk about a thousand negotiated moments.

## DOMESTIC VIOLENCE

The environment can take up to 40 IQ points off a child. The picture is bleak. On broad figures taken from research in 12 regional preschools in 2004, we estimated that about 70 percent of preschool Aboriginal children have experienced or witnessed domestic violence. The teachers queried our estimates; they thought perhaps as many as 90 percent of their children had been exposed to violence at home. Many children, instead of having a safe place to play at home, hear loud noises, mothers yelling, or worse, mothers drunk and numbed out of their minds, and fathers if present, mad on drugs, and witness violence, physical assaults. This has often been caused by influences from nonindigenous society into Aboriginal society, which seriously impacts abusive behavior from mothers and fathers. Domestic violence is born of despair and a terrible frustration that has no release except to attack what is loved, a violation of spirit that carries a murderous intensity in its response, frustration that has no answer in a war in which we are definitely the losers.

Hate is turned on partners, children, themselves. Harmony is lost, a particular vital emotional safe holding space is lost.

Terrible events such as domestic violence that confuse and confound are beyond a little child's sensitive awareness to grasp. The space that should be free to fantasize and dream is in a state of numbed fear from a horrible reality. This space is lost when it is intruded on by the imposition of violence on, and the violation of, the precious loved people in our world upon whom our security depends and, even worse, sometimes when violence is turned directly on the child. The space is lost when the parent has no space in their mind to hold the infant or little child. The child becomes no longer sacred, it is "thingified," and that means seen as an object available for the person's own pleasure not the child's need. This terrible reality forms a paradigm for all emotional distress created by the awareness or witnessing or being part of domestic violence and sexual abuse. If the intrusion is sexual, we speak of soul murder. What do children lose in such a situation? A sense of connectedness with themselves, a sense of connectedness with their family, a sense of connectedness with their community.

Children lose the capacity to fantasy, the capacity to play, and there in nothing in their life they can take for granted. There is a book by Judy Atkinson called *Beyond Violence: Finding Our Dream* (1990). Dreaming or fantasying is impossible in the wake of the dreadful impingement of the reality of violence. The fear is that something terrible will happen. The fear is that the child will fall into this terrible void created by trauma and lose its identity and secure base. That is the central fear of alcoholics and drug users, that they will fall into the pain and never make their way out again. So, they keep taking stuff to keep them up, up. We know that it is the sharing and witnessing of pain that allows for a cure.

> We cannot pretend it is not there or that it is harmless, we must absolutely acknowledge problems such as family violence, because we take responsibility and accept accountability in our search for solutions then. These solutions then become ours. There can be no true self-determination while the self remains unhealed. . . . Childhood trauma, abuse and neglect are a fundamental public health challenge—this is now widely recognized. And the challenge can be largely met with appropriate prevention and intervention . . . As a grandmother I could not live and think that I was handing to my grandchildren this legacy . . . That what had happened in our communities now—where violence has been normalized. (Atkinson 1990, 32)

## CASE: SAM

The director reported that Sam, a boy of three, was not going well. He was acting out more, and was destructive toward the other children's play and sometimes violent with them. Sam's mother Martha had arrived that morning and told Sam's teacher that she had had an abortion. Martha had talked freely about it in front of Sam. She said, "I'm 40 years of age, you'd think I would have learnt how to look after myself by now. Imagine getting pregnant and having to have an abortion." The staff would have liked to believe that Sam didn't understand, although he was standing with his mother the whole time.

When the play worker arrived at the discussion group to present her session with him she had no idea that Sam's mother had had an abortion, and was amazed by the revelation made after she presented her session with Sam. She reported,

> When I approached Sam, he saw that I had his play box and knew this was his special time. He came straight to me and decided that what he wanted to play with this morning were the little plastic bears. There are about 30 small baby and bigger adult bears, all the same shape and color. He took two bears, telling me, "This is a mummy bear and a baby bear," and he put them in a box which was open on the side. He got a hard covered book to use as a blocking wall on the box. I asked, "What are you doing?" and he said, "I'm making the mummy and baby bear safe from all the bad bears outside." He got all the rest of the bears out of the container, put them outside the box, and said, "See, they want to attack the mummy and the baby bear." Then with violently aggressive stamping he tried to crush the other bears. He told me, "These are very naughty bears they want to attack and kill the mummy's baby and the mummy too. I have to stop them." (Excerpt from case notes)

The group was stunned, thinking it extraordinary that Sam should be so conscious of the protection of the mother and baby at a time when the mother had aborted a baby. Did he fear to be aborted? we asked. How aware was this three-and-a-half-year-old child?

Later that week, the play worker reported:

> I observed the children queued up taking turns jumping from a springboard to a box, with the space between the board and the box widening each turn. All the other children could cope and enjoy it, but Sam could not. He was obviously terrified he would fall in the space between. I put the box as close to the board as he felt comfortable to jump. That was right alongside the board, with no gap between.

In this play Sam was revealed as an extremely frightened little boy: death was too close, and one could fall into the abyss, the space between too easily.

## ABSENCE, LOSS AND ABANDONMENT

Ninety percent of the Aboriginal children attending preschools in our regional area in 2004 had an absent father. This may have changed over time, although discussions with present-day teachers in Aboriginal preschools confirm suggest this figure may still be true. Even if it is half that number, it is still very serious. "Where have all the men gone?" Hiding in shame and numbed by drugs and alcohol—two suicides in the one family six months apart, and at exactly the same place. A respected elder calls me on the day of a funeral. She talks and cries for an hour on the phone. I cannot hang up. I have to let her cry, and I have to take the pain. She tries at first to escape by saying, "Foul play at hand and I will get those murderers who gave him the drugs." She finishes by saying, sadly and now quietly resigned, "He is his own killer. Why?"

There is mourning in a culture where loss on loss continues. That brilliant report "Bringing Them Home" (Human Rights and Equal Opportunity Commission 1997) makes horrific reading. I spoke at a conference:

> Where was home, who was mother? How dare we tell them, "Little children are sacred." Is that what we taught them as we took their children? We would bring them up to be servants, to be sexually abused by white bosses. Did we treat them as sacred, or you, the parent as sacred? We are sorry we took what was sacred to you and supplanted it with what was cultural and so-called superior to us. We robbed your children of family, culture, community. In almost every single case a parent was absent. The father protector was missing. When Ken Wyatt spoke at the Mental Health Conference (in Sydney, 2006) of how the men must stand by their women, he put his finger on the one significant weak point that leaves this culture unprotected. The absent father.

## THE UNPROTECTED CHILD

Why are children in orphanages or in institutions abused? Is it possible that when there is a lack of internal protective parents, the message given out is that this is an unprotected child, available to be used for one's selfish needs. The absence of a parent creates the presence of an abuser. The incredible demands placed on carers in the absence of a parent leaves the situation open to all sorts of abuse. It all goes back to a good internal and loving parent. When psychoanalysis began, Freud thought that the instinct was the center from which all flowed. Klein shone the torch on internal objects and saw this as the center—the internal battle acted out between good and bad spirits, and one might say and how these battles were fought and lost or won. Bion started the idea of a new basis, a basis from which something within us, not exactly known to us, called "the ineffable unknown," thought our thoughts, did our dreaming. Without a thinker, thoughts come to a bad end, become perverted, destructive, and undeveloped. This is the paradigm of the unprotected child. Is this what is happening, people who kill their own thoughts, their own value, their own life meaning, who survive but with a terrible survival that means killing the other? How does this happen?

## CASE: SERENA, WILL AND THE STORY OF A THREE-YEAR-OLD

Will, the father, sleeps in a bunk above his fourteen-year-old son's bed. He and his wife Serena are in therapy. His wife asks, "So why doesn't he take the space in my bed?" Will looked like he had got an electric shock; such a thought as taking or asserting his place was unknown to him. It is the father that teaches the son to demand, to assert, to have rights, to deserve respect. Will didn't have his father there when he was a child to teach him this. He taught him that the only way you can be yourself was to free yourself from the woman, by leaving and never returning, which he did when Will was three years old.

A child cannot play with an absent father. The child without a father cannot play. Will calls me, although it is his partner I see. He is going to leave if she does not treat his mother better. Three weekends later, Will walks out, telling me on the phone that she had robbed him of his adolescence and friends and life, and her jealous possessiveness was choking the life from him. Serena thinks he left despite every effort she made to be good, including coming to see me. For her, in the end everything, everyone dies. "You are left and at the end, you are just an abandoned piece of shit." She could not see that her insecurity made her cling so tightly she was choking him?

Thoughts began of the idea of an internal "obstructive object" that kills links, that kills thought, that deadens all imagination and dreaming.

Serena is a total mess, hyperventilating, having massive anxiety attacks, crying that she had never been loved all her life. She said Will was trying to remove her mother from their family. She needed her mother to exist, she told me. Will strongly resented Serena's mother, there was no room for him. Her mother ate up all the space. Serena hated his mother. Serena called his mother an interfering "c . . . ," and said his mother was all too available to have him back home with her. This is true, but it's not our concern here. We are interested in the little child, a girl just three years old.

The little child lay on the floor screaming, "I want my daddy! I want my daddy!" for hours on end. She had not eaten for two days. Her mother is now past the screaming and yelling and excited stage, she is in silent mourning.

"In my head I am hanging there with a strap around my neck. There is no other way out. The image haunts me day and night. I cannot cry any more. I am all washed out. I know now I'm a nothing!"

Will says, "I feel free like I am out of jail when I leave you. Nothing I ever do is good enough. You treat my mother like shit!" Stuff everywhere, no room, no space. She won't give him his things. She cannot bear the intolerable pain of losing him. He gets the police in. They stand protective witness as she is humiliated, destroyed and powerless again. Little girl lies on the floor. She cries and cries. She screams and screams—powerless also. In the end they have to physically restrain her. Her brother, who is fourteen, says to her, "We want him, but he doesn't want us anymore." Rage and hurt vie for supremacy in his tall powerful young frame. "He doesn't want us," he screams at her. His fourteen-year-old mind is enraged.

The twelve-year-old girl . . . beautiful, a life full of promise, a scholarship to one of the best schools, popular and loved by parents and peers. She cries and cries, refusing to go out anywhere. Day and night she cries. Her mother lets her sleep in her bed, so they comfort each other. The little three-year-old sleeps between them, having cried herself to sleep every night.

Every evening is the same. "I want my daddy! I want my daddy! Don't let the crocodile eat me." The twelve-year-old would call him to tell him her little sister was inconsolable. Sometimes he would come home and sit with her. He would comfort her. He would wait until she slept and then leave.

The little girl cannot, does not eat. She looks numb and is no more the happy free child I observed before. It's like all joy has left her. The mother is screaming, rude unbelievable words are screamed all over the neighborhood from my clinic room. Then I see she actually has no words underneath. It has the quality of a loud nothingness. She has no power. I show her this. She sees her own impotence. It shocks her. I show her how everything she says to her partner are threats and ultimatums, which just drive him away. She cannot ask for him. She cannot let him know her need of him. She is crying for him, and yet doing the very things that disempowered him and drove him away. She leaves that session thinking. Within a week he is back home and much more involved in the relationship than before.

I was left with a whole lot of questions: Can we only murder if we have already murdered ourselves? What part of us closes down so that we have no idea of the impact of our actions on the other? Will damages the people he loves unknowingly and yet in part of him he knows, someone in there knows. I am sure he comes home to save that child. How do we murder without knowing we are murdering? "Father forgive them, they know not what they do" has got to be the most powerful words. How can anyone forgive ignorance of this profound nature? My mind moves to the stolen generation. How did those people take the children from their parents, with the mother screaming and the children screaming, every bond of attachment ripped apart in a way that was mind-blowing in the anguish it created, and yet they knew not what they did. Why did Will leave? Was it because that part of him was already dead? Was it that the only way he could stop it from coming to life was to pass it on to another? His father had left, never to return, when Will was the age his daughter was now. Has that got something to do with it? Did he need her to know his pain or him to know his pain through her?

How does the childcare center, long-day stay or preschool help and support the traumatized child, parent, community, staff to survive and to cope with this enormous task?

## CARING FOR THE TEACHERS

So, who takes care of the teachers while the teachers take care of the children? The teachers do themselves! Staff need to take care of themselves to avoid burnout. A supportive family life helps, space to play themselves helps, not overworking helps. Being with young children in this sensitive state of development and trauma demands an openness to listening and supporting and encouraging that is incredibly exhausting. Teachers need debriefing and support. They need someone to talk to. They need supportive workshops. They need a sympathetic Board. They need not to be used and abused. They need a good wage. They need acknowledgement of the good work they do. The traumatized child touches a depth of emotion in carers that exposes their own trauma. Providing debriefing for the staff in a childcare center is the role of the director, supported by the Board.

So how do we do this when our own space is cluttered with rules, due process and governance, and there just is no time? How can we create a space for our charges when we do not have that space for ourselves? We have a paradox here—we are the best people to know and look after our own, we are the ones that know of our background, of our losses, and this makes us invaluable in helping our own children. This is an Aboriginal childcare center, they are our own and we are community. But what if we are suffering ourselves? What if our own pain is opened by their pain, what if our space is so cluttered with domestic violence and hurt that we do not have the mind-space ourselves? What if all our own dreams have turned to nightmares? How do we help our children to dare to dream? This is why we professionals must learn to trust each other and develop groups and boundaries where we can share and neutralize our pain and trauma. All too often, the dominance of the white fella has taught us a culture of power and we think we are above the parents or the children. What makes any center work is the commitment of staff and their support of each other. In our research, mothers liked it "that most of the staff are Indigenous and they like seeing the same known faces when they come in." They like you to use their name to greet them, they like to see you enjoying their children and involved in their children. The culture of domination and power must die as the powerless experience more power.

Training professional staff means supporting and hearing about their work with the children, hearing their traumas, and allowing expression of them, so they no longer suffer the sense of shame that trauma brings.

## KNOWING AND RESPECTING CULTURAL HERITAGE

Indigenous presence, whether it is created through family, mob, staff and other Indigenous involvement in the preschool, or an environment that is rich with Indigenous culture, is fundamental to providing a place where Indigenous children learn, and want to keep learning. It is a vital factor in making Indigenous children feel welcomed and valued in formal education.

*Chapter 12*

# The Unspeakable Nature of Trauma

In this chapter, I write about transgenerational trauma, the effect of a dead mother in infancy, which can create unspeakable trauma for the deadened child through into adulthood. Judy K. Eekhoff, to whom I owe much for extending and challenging and also validating my thinking around working with very distressed or disturbed patients, writes: "Ferenczi, Klein, Bion, as well as [Herbert] Rosenfeld attempted to treat and heal patients who suffered from early childhood traumas and who were in various stages of recovery from them. All came to believe that if the patient is to heal, the analyst must be willing to go to the depth of her own infantile trauma, and face the terror and rage of being a helpless and vulnerable infant, as well as splitting into the 'other' who was an observer of that trauma" (Eekhoff 2019, 71). She writes of a subjective experience of watching one's infantile self suffer to the point of breakdown.

I am using this thinking to make sense of what happened to me in my work with Jen. What happens to the internal psyche of an infant is hard to imagine, as he/she calls and calls for a mother and is not heard. The further traumatization by a stepfather's sexual intrusion on her at the age of eleven confirmed a deep adult disturbance. Adult patients who were as infants or as children psychically separated from their mother seem to be in a space where they do not psychically exist.

## CASE: JEN

Silence played a significant part in Jen's treatment. For two years of the therapy, neither she nor I could speak a word. Jen was referred to me by a pediatrician who was training as a child psychiatrist. He had referred her for therapy pertaining to postnatal depression. There were terrible unknowable silences in Jen's inner world. Later Jen described the silence as "unspeakable pain." There was the silence of her Jewish mother, interned during the Second World War. Not one word was ever spoken, nor did the children dare to ask what had happened to her during those war years. She could not ever speak about them. Until she died, if anything came on the radio to do with Germany, there was an enormous reaction and the radio was immediately turned off. She died well over ninety, and had still not spoken one word of her trauma during that time. Jen does not know if the Germans had killed her grandparents, but she does know her mother's silence was a known fact during her entire life.

Jen's first boyfriend was an Irish Catholic who was deeply and sincerely devoted to her. She was only seventeen, and she left him feeling he was not a good fit. She had sex with her second boyfriend, became pregnant, and had an abortion. This event began a conspiracy of silence, and neither she nor her mother ever mentioning it again. As a young adult she had gone to visit her father's brother's family in the United States at his invitation. She had an affair lasting several months with her uncle who was much younger than her father. She had no idea she was Jewish or even what Jewish meant, since she had been brought up Catholic, and her family name was a very common English name, which her stepfather adopted for the whole of his life. Aged eighteen as she was about to get on the plane to go and meet her uncle, her mother said, "I need to tell you that you are Jewish!" For the seventeen hours on the plane, she had pondered the meaning of this, another silence.

The real breakdown for her came, when happily married to Will, she had a miscarriage with her first pregnancy. She saw this as a punishment from God, both for her abortion and her sexually abusive relationship with her stepfather. Even though she abhorred her stepfather and the sexual abuse was against her will, she felt guilty.

In those early days of working with Jen, when she had two little children, I was aware of an enormous depression. She had a strong desire to move out of this, but nothing seemed to work. I could say she was totally absorbed in the children but being with them gave her no joy and much anxiety. They were very bright, lively children, but this only taxed her more and emphasized how depressed she was. Her son, who was like a hurricane, would bang his head in rage over and over on the concrete until it bled. The husband's total neglect of her and the children, working seven days a week and not at all relating to his daughter, made it harder.

Jen finally talked about her parents: "It was many years before I even got anything like a history about my mother's background, but I did know she had been in an internment camp for women in France and her husband had been in the camp for males in the same area." He was Jewish, but there was a strong English part of his family, and she had married him because he had an

English passport. They went to the English relatives after the war. He came to Australia to set up for her and his children, with the grandmother to come, but when Jen's mother arrived, he had no money, no job and no intention of bringing his mother to Australia. She described him as a womanizer who lived off the women with whom he had relationships.

When Jen was two years of age, her mother married her second husband and they had three children together. He was a brutal uncaring man, but the mother remained with him and "had to be grateful" to him, since their survival as a unit was impossible without his presence. He interfered sexually with Jen, beginning when she was ten and up to the age of fourteen, which coincided with three pregnancies her mother had during this time. When she got her periods, he was disgusted and called her a "dirty filthy girl," but still approached her. Aged 15, her mother and sister went on a holiday. He approached her while they were away. She told him if he ever came near her again, she would tell her mother, the police and anyone who would listen. I began to wonder how her mother did not know what was going on. Jen reported that the mother found out during her adolescence, when Jen's sister screamed at her mother in rage, that she was leaving home because of what her stepfather had done to her. It was then that Jen realized he had been also abusing her sister. The sister left home at sixteen, never to return, but has remained close to Jen, seeing her almost every day. It must have been well into a year in the therapy when Jen started to tell me about her own childhood, and her mother and father's background. I met her sister at Jen's husband's funeral 46 years later, and she came and thanked me, which gave me the impression that she had used very well what Jen had taken from her work with me. She said, "Thank you for saving my sister's life. I know who you are."

As Jen began to improve, it became obvious that she needed a full analytic therapy. She chose to stay sitting up and was absolutely against lying down. I wondered if this was linked to her not being able to trust lying down, as it would leave her exposed and vulnerable. When Jen agreed to change the nature of the therapy, her material, or I should say the lack of material, became central to the entire process. She would acknowledge me in the waiting room, greeting me with a nod, and then enter the room where no contact would be made for the entire session. She would sit and look, as if transfixed, glazed over, not present. I have to say the supervision around this time held me, even as I held her. We decided it was very important to go through this stage she was in, not intruding on it in any way. I had no idea how long it would last, and it began to become more difficult for me to tolerate the sessions. I would wake up in the morning dreading that it was the day I had to go through this with Jen. I knew it had to be done. My own mind began to lose itself, my thinking became confused; I was lost in an autistic-like space that seemed to have no resolution. The only thing that held me was my supervisor, and faith in the process. It became harder with each session, and it's hard to believe that it went on for nearly two years. I would leave the session, go inside, and crouch in the corner of a room, holding my head in both hands until my thinking returned. What must this child have suffered? What unbearable autistic space was she inviting me to know and understand with her? Tustin (1990b, 132) wrote, "The feeling of brokenness goes to the very fabric of their being . . . their sense of being was felt to be threatened. Annihilation stared them in the face, and very desperate steps had to be taken to combat it. To combat it and to cover their brokenness, they developed the plaster cast of autism. This concretized experience of encapsulation spells death to the psyche . . . Understanding their sense of agony helps us."

Finally. in that second year, something happened inside me and I knew I could not stand it anymore without giving it words. But how was I to give it words without intruding on her space, or trying to force her out of it in any way? I suggested to my supervisor that I might just trial a soliloquy, in which I would talk, not looking at her, but looking at the wall. I told her what I was going to do, and it seemed as if she didn't hear me. I began to talk about how she experienced that space as a whole empty nothingness, "a nowhere, no one, nothing happening" space. This was the central core of her trauma, this autistic space, where nothing could be thought or known, because it was unthinkable and unknowable. I had to know it, she had to know I knew it. The soliloquy, a kind of talking, seemed not to intrude, and I doubted she even heard it. One day many sessions later, I said, "The powerlessness, the sense of being a victim with no control, the child maybe died and maybe you can't tell me the child inside you is dead. You cannot even go into the space of the atrocities that killed the child." One day in the midst of my talking like this, she spoke, "No you have that wrong! The child isn't dead, it's alive, but it doesn't know how to tell the adult that it's alive." These were the first words spoken in two years, and I was stunned. She just talked on, but briefly in a very ordinary way.

Gradually over the sessions, the blackness, the raging anger, the unmitigated hatred towards the intruder took over. Eekhoff (2019, 90) writes about how impulse is restored in therapy and how "with impulse comes turmoil when coming alive is terrifying and enraging. Coming alive can be so terrifying it traumatizes the patient again." However, Jen began to recover, and one of the joys was going to a class where she learnt sculpturing, which she developed to a very professional level. The pieces were exquisite. The words she spoke in sessions were chosen carefully and beautifully presented, but one could see she was alive and well. Sometime later she finished the therapy, and I expected not to see her again. I was therefore very surprised when she presented some ten years later and was in a highly anxious and confused state, and feeling that she was losing her mind. What made it worse was that no amount of therapy appeared to make her feel any better, and indeed she seemed to be getting worse, which made no sense at all. One day I asked her if she would go and have a complete physical check, as I could see no emotional reason for the way she was. She was found to have a severe thyroid problem and was put on medication which took some time to get adjusted for her. The endocrinologist understood that her childhood may well have been a contributory factor. Whatever the cause, she made a good recovery, and after a year of therapy, I was not to see her again for many years.

## Years Later

Some twenty-five years later, she called me and came to see me, bringing her husband with her. "My husband is very ill. We both know he is dying. There is something I must do," and with this she took out a letter of several pages which she read to me. Her husband spoke volubly of his anger with her stepfather. She sent this letter to her stepbrothers and sisters, letting them know of the terrible tragic effects of their father's atrocities with her. Her husband was totally supportive, and it was hard to believe this kind and gentle man was the husband who seemed so absent for her over those years. She engaged him in a caring and loving way, and he was most responsive and caring. He died some months later. She requested I go to the funeral and asked if she could see me for the period after his death. I was glad to do this for her. Was her mother's unknowing of the sexual abuse because she could not, did not, face or resolve what had happened to her in that concentration camp? Did she unwittingly allow the same experience, of which she could not talk, to happen with both the children through the atrocity of sexual intrusion on their young selves? Jen thinks she was so switched off she did not think or know about protecting her girls. I have no answer to these questions. Nor do I know how much my patient's silence was her mother's silence, that which has no words, which doubts the possibility of words and the possibility of the words being heard.

> The essential element in the case of the psychically dead mother isn't a traumatic precocious interruption of the mother's presence by her real sudden death or separation, but that the child grows up in the presence of a mother absorbed in an inner world of blank bereavement, depression and deadness. The mother's blank mourning brings in the child a massive de-cathexis of the maternal object, resulting in a psychical hole in the texture of object relations with the mother. (Eshel 2019, 47)

I saw Jen for over a year after her husband died. It certainly was not analysis and appeared to me like a mourning any wife of fifty years would do. Her children were so supportive, and she had dinner each evening with her son and his wife and their three teenage children, all of whom loved her dearly, whom she drove to school and to the university. Her daughter, who lived 200 kilometers away, visited with her partner on weekends and telephoned daily.

## Discussion

Now there is a further issue in trauma that is not quite repetition so much as a continuity that crosses generations. The secrets revealed by Jen's mother became those unrevealed in her own life, to do with the stepfather, the pregnancy and abortion, the miscarriage. In her mind she made it very clear to me many years later they were all one of the same. Finally, the mind could no longer hold the degree of trauma imposed by this continuum, and there was no way at all for her to speak of them, to seek help with them, to believe that anyone would be able to hold them and be able to transform them in doses that were tolerable and bearable by her. This frozen, unmoving, internal world destroys the meaning in anything living. I write here of a madness the therapist must be able to enter in their own living experience in order to reach it in the patient. This madness that may not even be born of the patient's experience but that of a previous generation. She was aware of her mother's depression up to the day she died.

In *History Beyond Trauma* (2004), Davoine and Gaudillière (2004, 256) write of "frozen times and frozen trauma." In reality, this "bloody rough way" as Wittgenstein called it, "goes through traumas and madness to secure the production of freedom among men." For there was definitely proved livingness and health in this patient and it cost me enormously, but it was worth it to see Jen now living and enjoying being alive. In the final analysis, is it worth the investment, one might ask. The answer is undoubtedly "yes," it is.

*Chapter 13*

# The Transformational Process of Working Through Early Childhood Trauma in Adult Psychotherapy

This chapter focuses on the effects on the therapist of working with adult trauma that dates back to pregnancy, birth and early childhood. I present my clinical work with Michael, an infant life beginning with a traumatized and deadened mother. His therapy formed a very painful out-of-the-ordinary experience, remaining part of my psychic experience for years after his therapy concluded. How does trauma suffered by a parent become transgenerational trauma transmitted to a pregnancy, to the birth of an infant, influencing his psyche from its roots all through into adulthood? This is a narrative of therapeutic working from a deadened center in which I was deadened for two years, I experienced a psychotic-like mind-state during his sessions. I had autistic-like suffering in an extraordinary way, feeling stunned, immobilized, psychotic during the sessions, so that I needed time afterward to recover and restore my mind to a state of equilibrium.

I had many concerns. Did I have an inner psychic unresolved problem? Was I doing something therapeutically wrong? What was creating this total "wipe out" of both myself and my patient during his sessions over such a long period? Two things were important. One was the incredible motivation on the part of the patient to work and recover; the patient did not miss one session. The second was that I was supervised all the way through by a very skilled senior psychoanalyst, who helped me hold "faith" in the process. In the end it was hearing the patient that created the resolution. This patient did so well, I came to believe that this numbed or deadened experience was an important part of the process, preceding any links to being alive for the first time. Strangely, I saw him at work some forty years later and can attest to his living a meaningful and purposeful life. It was obvious how well his life had resolved. That allowing of life in a deadened center in trauma through three or four sessions a week over some ten years or more demonstrated the capacity of the human spirit to recover.

We can begin by presuming there was not only a dead mother, but a dead infant. When Winnicott wrote "there is no such thing as a baby," he was writing about how no infant can survive without a mother, and no mother can survive as a mother to that infant if the infant dies. There is a double mourning, but we are thinking here of the traumatized mother, not alive to her infant, and the infant then beginning life as if psychically dead. As I noted in the previous chapter, Eshel (2019, 47) writes how "the child grows up in the presence of a mother absorbed in an inner world of blank bereavement, depression and deadness." She says this brings about "in the child a massive de-cathexis of the maternal object resulting in a psychic hole," and this brings about not just, "the loss of love but a loss of meaning." She adds further that "it becomes for him forbidden to be." It was this powerful forbidding to be for the patient that was central, but I, as the therapist mother, was forbidden to be also. It was my daring to tolerate this that created its resolution.

Michael's years of attendance was marked by an enormous desire to escape out of this "forbidden to be" and to "become alive." The shattering of the at-oneness very early, I suspect before birth even, was followed by a childhood with further trauma. For the young male patient, separated from his mother at the age of three for nine months, sent to live with his grandparents while his mother was pregnant with twins, left him even more despairing and empty, their birth pushing him into a further sense of his own nothingness. Can such trauma be repaired and healed? As with Jen (see Chapter 12), in this case the patient and I were released to "be." I saw it not as a repair but as a new beginning. It felt like the Sunday of Easter, a vulnerable fragile egg-like new beginning, of incredible sensitivity, occurring between us both. There had been a new experience of the at-oneness, and with it a creating of a new life with an alive mother and an alive child. Bion (1977, 156) added "that transformations in O is a new experience that happens, that can only 'be' and 'become' but it cannot be known."

## CASE: MICHAEL

The death of a newborn profoundly influences later living infants, particularly the next. The vulnerability and sensitivity of previous loss strikes at the very core of relations between the mother and her infant if the death is not, and cannot be, processed. Michael, when referred for therapy, was a depressed man in his late thirties, who on having left the priesthood was working in a railway goods yard cleaning the showers and toilets of the railway employees.

He had been a priest in a city parish. He had doubts and struggles during that time in relating to the organization of the church and his place within it. The turning point came when he fell in love with an unmarried high school teacher. He was confused about the direction he should take in his own future life and career, and how he could resolve the conflict of being deeply in love with Sarah a Catholic teacher while remaining true to his vows as a priest. Although he was given leave from Church duties to resolve his own future choices, he could see no way of doing this. He took his vows most seriously. His entire work as a priest lost none of its in-depth spirituality. He still attended daily mass. His deep thinking, his capacity for contemplative prayer remain to this day. The unmarried teacher was equally in love with him and committed to him. He had not acted out his desires, nor had Sarah, while there was no resolution of the situation for either of them.

From the beginning he was articulate, deep thinking, willing to trust the nature of the work of therapy, and that trust was basic and unfailing through the years of realizing the depth of his problems. At its very core was his mother's failure, due to her own traumas, to experience him as separate from the baby who had died two days after birth, right before Michael was conceived. He was exactly one year older than his dead sibling and was given the exact male equivalent of her female name. His mother and father were genuinely devoted to each other, but during her first pregnancy there was a terrible accident at his father's workplace on the railways, where he was a shunter in the goods yard. A carriage had become uncoupled and ran down on him as he was working, severing his arm and resulting in amputation. This was an enormous blow to him and to their relationship as a couple, and the father lived the rest of his life with one arm.

Michael's mother's first pregnancy was uneventful, but the baby girl's death two days after birth was unresolved and deeply traumatizing. Soon after, his mother fell pregnant with him, her second child. The mother now with a dead baby and a husband with one arm removed was described by my patient as approaching psychosis. In this state she gave birth to a healthy baby boy. She called him by the male equivalent of his sister's name. Neither he nor I were sure she ever saw him as a separate child, but rather as the male equivalent of that first baby. Certainly, throughout his therapy he became more and more convinced that she never experienced him as himself; in his own mind, there was always confusion. He later was to say, he was not sure he ever existed in her mind as a separate person.

The early months and years in therapy were totally preoccupied with our analytic work, which he took very seriously. He knew he should resolve the journey of his life, but he stood at the fork in the road for some years, unsure how to resolve his dilemma. He knew he deeply loved the teacher, but felt emotionally dead and in a "dead end job" with no financial future. He was in an abyss where he felt no life or existence. He said, "How can I commit to give myself in a loving marital relationship when I do not feel I have a self to give." My work took on a stranger and stranger turn as I experienced myself as being there but not conscious, and if conscious not able to move. Something far more than the conflict of what to do with his life was being lived out. Where a core of self should have been was an empty autistic state so powerful that it took many months, maybe even years to resolve.

I began to dread the sessions, afraid that I might reveal the intense distortions in my own thoughts. The countertransference was crippling. I would sit crouched in a corner for an hour after his sessions until I regained my own mind. I became afraid I would express out loud my crazy random thoughts elicited by his presence. It was like a sleep or an awake kind of blurred nothingness. His presentation at this time was lost and my appearing asleep was bewildering to him. He later told me he just thought he was boring, and so I had fallen asleep. This was held by good supervision on my side, and Michael's capacity for steadfast resilience on his side, but it took us both through ensuing unutterable psychic pain. It took an enormous push of psychic strength to break through, holding the faith in what was an almost impossible non-faith time. It was at this time that a strange paradox was clear to me. It is only in the capacity to dare to have no faith that true faith is born. "Faith is not a comfort or a false raft to cling to, but a faith born in the no faith. Hope born where there was no hope, not as a comforting reassurance but as a light in the total darkness. Love was born where no love could be, in a loveless space. It was a gentle backwards and forwards movement in this that made up the movement and growth in the therapy" (Caputo 1987, 76).

Michael asked if he could share the writing of this chapter with me. Some 30 years after our initial sessions, Michael related this in this way:

> For two years I laid on that couch almost daily with nothing to say. I made a flying leap from the chair on to the couch, and absolutely nothing was going on in my mind and in my being. I was aware you also were in a stupor but eventually able to break through it, and somehow this communicated to me, and it was with each breakthrough from you, there was a breakthrough from me. I remember the feeling that as my infant trauma was exposed, the feeling was like being dropped through the gates of an emotional death. I could see how my mother's "psychotic" depression left me prematurely and permanently separated from her. It threw me into an abyss of annihilating nothingness. The relationship with my therapist was an invitation to enter into the abyss of unutterable suffering. Through contact with my therapist there is a part of me that was learning to be connected to life, an attempt to know and be attuned to the pain in the center of trauma, not the deadness, the terror of pain. My blocking it and all the emotional effects that I held within my own heart, blocked me from any chance of connecting human love to the "other." (Personal correspondence to author, 2021)

Looking on from outside, one could be deceived into seeing Michael's early life as nothing more than an ordinary suburban childhood, the exception being a long period with his grandparents when his mother was pregnant with twins when he was two years old. From the beginning he was an alone introverted child. That separation deeply disturbed him, adding to his trauma, and compounding it. Was he now no longer relevant, he asked himself, as the twins seemed to such a very young child to be his replacement? Was he ever alive or seen as alive? Was he mixed up so much with that first baby, he was her not him? Was he never born? These thoughts preoccupied him, not in any judgment of his mother, but as an effort to resolve something we named as an autistic core in his personality. It was not just a lesion, a wound, to him it was all pervading, total. There was no sense of being.

The work was difficult and slow with each dosage of minute pain. There was a sense of being alive to suffer it, as little by little he experienced himself as real. He held strongly to his faith with daily mass. As his therapy progressed, he decided to go to university to do social work, which seemed to him to be closest to his priestly work. The young "unknowingness" of the world around him was very clear, as he came in devastated when his first assignment mark was a D, which he saw to be close to a failure, thinking the marks went ABCDEF. When he went to see his lecturer to find out why he had done so badly, he was amazed to be told a D was for a distinction, and indeed he had a right to complain as his essay deserved an HD (high distinction), but the lecturer felt giving that for a first essay would leave no space for further essays to be marked up. His humility, which deepened into an even richer spirituality throughout his life, was the one enduring quality that seemed to mark his entire living experience.

After a long retreat and much searching, he finally took the leap into an enormous love of the teacher, the woman now to be his wife. He struggled with thoughts of whether he could love, give love, and be a worthy partner to this woman. She had waited patiently, understanding his journey all too well, since she had her own childhood traumas as an inmate of an orphanage from the age of three. After a thirty-day retreat, Michael made the decision to marry. After being knocked back for a period, the church gave him dispensation to leave the priesthood. Both he and his wife to be had no doubt of this as the right step, and the celebration and joy in it was profound. Her many friends and members of their faith celebrated with them, going to their wedding. He was satisfied that it was a love blessed by God, and although some of the senior priests emotionally condemned and abused him for leaving his "calling," he was steadfast in his holding and loyalty to his wife. He was in his final university year.

One day a year later I was amazed to receive a call from his wife, saying she knew she must not talk to me, but she was so proud of him, and he was too humble to tell me he had graduated with first class honors. He had left therapy at that time, and there was no contact with him. He began working as a social worker. Then at the end of their first year of marriage his wife was diagnosed with breast cancer. He returned to therapy at his request. The therapy focused on this living trauma that was beyond his belief. After all they had been through to find each other, the shock for both was horrendous. She also saw a therapist, known to Michael and myself during this time, working on the trauma that was beyond his belief. The cancer was treated with a lumpectomy and radiation. She remained well for six years, but just as it seemed safe to have hope the cancer returned. He returned once more to therapy. She had a breast removed and chemotherapy and was well until four years later when cancer returned once more. The couple battled for two years as she was dying.

His therapy at that time was of unbelievable love and sorrow. Grief consumed him, even while love made it possible to care for her in every way. They made precious visits to the mountains from the city where they lived. He told the story of their bathing together in the mountain retreat. There was no hope between them for her to live. He tried to talk about it. "We both sat in a bath together and I thought it was going to be a sensual experience, but what I found was that she was in another dimension of consciousness. When I thought about it afterward, it seemed to have significance of the rite of baptism, which is a rite into life, a rite into birth and death, since all that lives dies. It was a preparation for her death for her and me." The presence of a therapist became most relevant to hold him through this agonizing time. He spoke of walking to the very gate of death with her and saying "goodbye" there. He spoke of how her death, this loss, threw him into an emotional abyss of annihilating black grief that mirrored and opened into his traumatic infantile experience. Over time he could say at the end of therapy he felt that the abyss of death had been transformed into an abyss of life and love:

> I begin to have this sense of how can I understand my life? The basic belief of Buddha is that life is a journey of suffering. I began to think how my whole life has been preoccupied with the suffering of the initial trauma I had been born into. Intergenerational trauma from both my mother and father's family. There is a part in the gospel of Christ as a suffering servant who takes into himself the suffering of mankind, epitomized in the crucifixion. I experience myself as a suffering servant with the trauma of my own life, intersecting with my father and mother's family trauma. I was the one who held it within me, suffered it and was now able to dare to feel it and live that journey of suffering as a result of it. Therapy gave me a life I had not had, but it also gave me the capacity "to suffer the suffering in the suffering." There are two aspects here. It gave me the empathy to work with the trauma of others, but further to this is the knowledge that trauma is a sacred wound and that changes everything. I found my experience of

> the therapy process as my therapist inviting me to open my heart to love, a love that comes from the very depths of who I am. Because of trauma, that capacity to open my heart from the very core was blocked by the emotional trauma and its effect. Norma was attuned to the blockages that stopped me from opening my heart to life. Each time those blockages were resolved there was a transforming, a moment of a giving of myself, a moment of experiencing myself as alive to my therapist and therefore to the world. This openness was the opposite of that not daring to trust that seemed to be at the very core of my being. I had to dare to trust, and to risk being unknown, rejected or accepted. That is the transformation of trauma from deadness into a living experience, into the very core of who I am. (Personal correspondence to author, 2021)

For myself, as his therapist, I saw this transformation from being so blocked to a place now of symbolization and mysticism as part of the movement from the darkness of the abyss to light. If one can dare to wait in that dark space then the life will come from within, the "spark" as enunciated by Meister Eckhart. After trauma is resolved, the patient and therapist become not more like each other, but more like their selves, so that the introverted, deep thinking spiritual person uses his depth and his thinking, his spirituality in a far more creative fashion. There is something about spirituality in the therapy relationship that points to the particular quality that allows freedom of the other to emerge, to be themselves. The ultimate gift of therapy is that the person comes out of it truly grounded in their own core and their own uniqueness.

The sort of emotional space required in the therapy is one where the therapist empties themself of self, and is able to be totally there for the other in a way that allows the emergence of difference in the other to be born. Bion speaks about letting go of memory, understanding and desire. He is speaking of letting go of those realities in order to be self-emptying and other-centered. Creativity born out of trauma is not the healing of pain, but the capacity to suffer it, and through that is healing born, and with it a creative and meaningful life. The therapist has a place of unique tolerance and empathy, an emptying of self to allow the other the space to be themselves.

Some twenty years later, I wrote to Michael and asked his permission to use his case material in this chapter. He was pleased to grant it. He asked me if I could include the following passage in his chapter: he called it, "Confronting the Demonic Psychic Self."

> When I entered analytic therapy, I was struck with how emotionally enclosed and cut off I was in the initial two years. As the therapy progressed, I began to become aware of a terrifying persona in me to subvert and destroy any emergent new life of my traumatized infant self. I began to understand it as a demonic part of myself, because its sole objective seemed to be to direct its hatred towards

any emergent new life energy. At times I felt it actually enjoy crushing any new life energy. As I reflect back, I understood it more clearly through the scientists discovering the black hole in our galaxy. The black hole that drags in stars, planets, gas dust into oblivion, struck me as an analogy for this destructive anti-life force in me. It seemed to gain its power through "sucking up" the psychic energy of unconscious from my un-suffered traumatic wounding. I discovered Dante's poem of Virgil traversing Hell, Purgatory and Heaven as a wonderful way of understanding my "trauma journey." Hell is the psychic space where the wound of trauma un-suffered grows in power and intensity and destructiveness the longer it is left unattended; Purgatory is the process of release into the suffering of the trauma; Heaven is the new life that emerges out of the experienced wound. This tripartite traumatic wound in this framework is also potentially a sacred wound that connects me to the ground of my being, with all its creative energy of love, compassion, wisdom and mercy. (Personal correspondence to author, 2021)

# *Chapter 14*

# And in the End

As I was coming to the end of writing this book, I had a very strange dream, which puzzled me at first. I dreamt my four-year-old daughter had died. The shock of finding her dead awakened me in fright. I did not have a daughter, but looking more closely, I saw it was my four-year-old self, who had been traumatized by an abrupt and terrible separating from my family at that age. Guided by our "Dream Group" with whom I shared this dream, I had insight into one of the most important psychic processes in healing trauma. I realised the psychic death at the core of trauma cannot be restored to life. "When you're dead, you're dead!" What, then, is the treatment of trauma about? From whence comes the healing? The healing of trauma is in the experiencing of mourning for the death of the self, from the internal implosion occurring in trauma. That is what the good-enough therapist, the good enough family, the good enough community does to heal trauma. And the second part is something like this, to dare with the presence of a holding "other" to face the unbearable suffering of loss, to sit in the darkness, not striving for the light. It means not grabbing external light in whatever form, self-glorification or brilliance, but being resigned to the death of self, caused by trauma, waiting in the darkness until the spark comes, from within. That is life after trauma. That is life vulnerable at first, but in the end full of possibilities. The real recovery, from whence is born true giftedness, is the capacity to wait in the inner darkness of loss for the spark, the gift "from within." Some people call it "God" or "spirit" inside of us.

Too easy to only call it manic or narcissistic, as indeed omnipotence is one of the defenses against trauma. But this is a true gift for the traumatized who experience healing. It makes them ordinary, by allowing them the gift of being, of being alive again in humility and without a sense of omnipotence. In one of many follow-up studies of the child soldiers in Rwanda, those who went back to their village and were accepted actually grew up with remarkable gifts of leadership and resilience. Those who had no family, or no village to return to, went to the cities and became remarkable as murderers and thieves. The transformational quality in the healing of trauma is love, not gooey sentimental love, but true holding love, the empathy that the therapist brings to the patient, that the family brings to one of their own, that the “mob” brought to the ancient Aboriginal in the performing of Dadirri.

# References


Ainsworth Mary, Mary Blehar, Everett Waters, and Sally Wall. 1978. *Patterns of Attachment: A Psychological Study of the Strange Situation*. Hillsdale, NJ: Erlbaum.

Atkinson, Judy. 1990. *Beyond Violence: Finding Our Dream*. Canberra: The Aboriginal and Islander Sub-program, National Domestic Violence Education Program, Office of Status of Women.

———. 2002. *Trauma Trails, Recreating Song Lines: The Transgenerational Effects of Trauma in Indigenous Australia*. Melbourne: Spinifex Press.

Badura-Brack, Amy, Timothy J. McDermott, Elizabeth Heinrichs-Graham, Tara J. Ryan, Maya M. Khanna, Daniel S. Pine, Yair Bar-Haim, and Tony W. Wilson. 2018. "Veterans with PTSD Demonstrate Amygdala Hyperactivity While Viewing Threatening Faces: a MEG study." *Biological Psychology* 132: 228–32.

Benedek, Therese. 1952. *Psychosexual Functions in Women*. New York: Ronald Press.

Bibring, Grete L. 1959. "Some Considerations of the Psychological Processes in Pregnancy." *The Psychoanalytic Study of the Child* 14 (1): 113–21.

Bibring, Grete L., Thomas F. Dwyer, Dorothy S. Huntington, and Arthur F. Valenstein. 1961. "A Study of the Psychological Processes in Pregnancy and of the Earliest Mother-Child Relationship: II. Methodological Considerations." *The Psychoanalytic Study of the Child* 16 (1): 25–44.

Bick, Esther. 1968. "The Experience of the Skin in Early Object-Relations." *International Journal of Psychoanalysis* 49 (2–3): 484–86.

Bion, Wilfred. 1957. "Differentiation of the Psychotic from the Non-Psychotic Personalities." *International Journal of Psychoanalysis*, 38: 266–75.

———. 1962. *Learning from Experience*. London: Heinemann.

———. 1963. *Elements of Psycho-Analysis*. London: Heinemann.

———. 1965. *Transformations: Change from Learning to Growth*. London: Heinemann.

———. 1977. *Seven Servants: Four Works*. Lanham, MD: Jason Aronson.

Bollas, Christopher. 1987. *The Shadow of the Object: Psychoanalysis of the Unthought Known*. London: Free Association Books.

Bowlby, John. 1969. *Attachment and Loss, Volume 1: Attachment*. London: Hogarth Press and The Institute of Psychoanalysis.

———. 1973. *Attachment and Loss: Volume 2: Separation.* London: Hogarth Press and The Institute of Psychoanalysis.

Brazelton, T. Berry. 1988. "Preparing for Parenthood." Unpublished paper delivered at NSW Institute of Psychotherapy, Sydney. Talk recorded by the author, and used by permission

Brazelton, T. Berry, and Bertrand G. Cramer. 1990. *The Earliest Relationship: Parents, Infants, and the Drama of Early Attachment*. Boston, MA: Addison-Wesley.

Caputo, John. 1987. *Radical Hermeneutics: Repetition, Deconstruction, and the Hermeneutic Project*. Bloomington: Indiana University Press

———. 2001. *On Religion*. London: Routledge.

Charles, Marilyn. 2014. "Trauma, Fragmentation, Memory, and Identity." In *Fragments of Trauma and the Social Production of Suffering: Trauma, History, and Memory*, edited by Michael O'Loughlin and Marilyn Charles, 25–44. Lanham, MD: Rowman & Littlefield.

Cohn, Jeffrey, and Edward Tronick. 1983. "Three-month-old Infant's Reaction to Simulated Maternal Depression." *Child Development* 54 (1): 185–93.

Cowan, James. 1994. *Myths of The Dreaming: Interpreting Aboriginal Legends*. Santa Rosa, CA: Atrium Publishers Group.

Davoine, Francoise, and Jean-Max Gaudillière. 2004. *History Beyond Trauma*. Translated by Susan Fairfield. New York: Other Press.

De Monchaux, Cecily. 1962. "Thinking and Negative Hallucination." *International Journal of Psychoanalysis* 43: 311–14.

Department of Employment Education Training and Youth Affairs. 2000. *National Indigenous English Literacy and Numeracy Strategy 2000–2004*. Canberra: Commonwealth of Australia.

Deutsch, Helene. 1945. *The Psychology of Women, Volume 2: Motherhood.* New York: Grune and Stratton.

Eaton, Jeff. 2011. "The Obstructive Object." In *A Fruitful Harvest: Essays After Bion*, 17–33. Seattle, WA: Alliance Press.

Eckhart, Meister. 1981. *The Essential Sermons, Treatises, Commentaries and Defense*, translated by Edmund Colledge and Bernard McGinn. New York: Paulist Press.

———. 2001. *Wandering Joy: Meister Eckhart's Mystical Philosophy*, translated by Reiner Schürmann. Great Barrington, MA. Lindisfarne Books.

Eekhoff, Judy K. 2019. *Trauma and Primitive Mental States: An Object Relations Perspective*. London and New York: Routledge.

Eigen, Michael. 1985. "Towards Bion's Starting Point: Between Catastrophe and Faith." *International Journal of Psychoanalysis*, 66 (3): 321–30.

———. 1993. *The Electrified Tightrope*, edited by Adam Phillips. Northvale, NJ: Jason Aronson.

———. 2004a. *Psychic Deadness*. London: Karnac Books.

———. 2004b. *The Psychotic Core*. London: Karnac Books.

———. 2006. "The Annihilated Self." *Psychoanalytic Review* 93 (1): 25–38.

Eshel, Ofra. 2019. *The Emergence of Analytic Oneness: Into the Heart of Psychoanalysis*. London and New York: Routledge.

Farrelly, Eileen. 2003. *Dadirri: The Spring Within: The Spiritual Art of the Aboriginal People from Australia's Daly River Region*. Darwin, Australia: Terry Knight and Associates.

Feder, Luis. 1980. "Preconceptive ambivalence and external reality." *International Journal of Psychoanalysis* 61 (2): 161–78.

Field, Tiffany, Miguel Diego, and Maria Hernandez-Reif. 2010. "Preterm Infant Massage Therapy Research: A Review." *Infant Behavior & Development* 33 (2): 115–124.

Flood, Josephine. 2006. *The Original Australians: Story of The Aboriginal People*. Crows Nest: Allen & Unwin.

Fonagy, Peter, Miriam Steele, George Moran, Howard Steele, and Anna Higgitt. 1992. "Measuring the Ghost in the Nursery: An Empirical Study of the Relation between Parents' Mental Representations of Childhood Experiences and Their Infants' Security of Attachment." *Journal of the American Psychoanalytic Society* 41 (4): 957–89.

Freud, Sigmund. 1957a. "On Narcissism: An Introduction (1914)." In *The Standard Edition of the Complete Psychological Works of Sigmund Freud, Volume XIV (1914–1916): On the History of the Psycho-Analytic Movement, Papers on Metapsychology and Other Works*, edited by James Strachey, 67–102. London: Hogarth Press.

———. 1957b. "Mourning and Melancholia (1917)." In *The Standard Edition of the Complete Psychological Works of Sigmund Freud, Volume XIV (1914–1916): On the History of the Psycho-Analytic Movement, Papers on Metapsychology and Other Works*, edited by James Strachey, 237–58. London: Hogarth Press.

———. 1963. "Lecture XVIII: Fixation to Traumas—The Unconscious." In *The Standard Edition of the Complete Psychological Works of Sigmund Freud, Volume XVI (1916–1917): Introductory Lectures on Psycho-Analysis (Part III)*, edited by James Strachey, 273–285. London: Hogarth Press.

———. 1966. "Extracts from the Fleiss Papers: Draft A." In *The Standard Edition of the Complete Psychological Works of Sigmund Freud, Volume I (1886–1899): Pre-Psycho-Analytic Publications and Unpublished Drafts*, edited by James Strachey, 177–78. London: Hogarth Press.

———. 1995. "The Interpretation of Dreams." In *The Basic Writings of Sigmund Freud*, Translated and edited by Abraham Brill, 149–520. New York: The Modern Library.

García Badaracco, Jorge. 1992. "Psychic Change and its Clinical Evaluation." *International Journal of Psychoanalysis* 73 (2): 209–20.

Garner, Paul. 2000. "Listening to the Space between Life and Death." In *Parents of Premature Infants: Their Emotional World*, edited by Norma Tracey. London: Whurr.

Green, André. 1986. *On Private Madness*. London: Hogarth Press.

Grinberg, Leon. 1990. *The Goals of Psychoanalysis: Identification, Identity and Supervision*. London: Karnac Books.

Grotstein, James. 2000. *Who Is the Dreamer Who Dreams the Dream? A Study of Psychic Presences*. Hillsdale, NJ: Analytic Press.

Guntrip, Harry. 1968. *Schizoid Phenomena, Object-Relations, and the Self.* London: Hogarth Press and the Institute of Psychoanalysis

Harris, Martha. 2011. "Some Notes on Maternal Containment in 'Good Enough' Mothering [1975]." In *The Tavistock Model: Papers on Child Development and Psychoanalytic Training*, by Martha Harris and Esther Bick, 139–60. London: Karnac Books.

Hedges, Lawrence. 1994. *In Search of the Lost Mother of Infancy*. New York: Jason Aronson.

Heidegger. Martin. 1982. *Nietzsche: Volume Four: Nihilism*, edited by David Krell. New York: Harper & Row.

Human Rights and Equal Opportunity Commission. 1997. *Bringing Them Home: Report of the National Inquiry into the Separation of Aboriginal and Torres Strait Islander Children from Their Families*. Canberra: Commonwealth of Australia

Isaacs, Jennifer, comp. ed. 2005. *Australian Dreaming: 40,000 Years of Aboriginal History*. Sydney, Australia: New Holland.

Joseph, Betty. 1981. "Towards the Experiencing of Psychic Pain." In *Do I Dare Disturb the Universe? A Memorial to W. R. Bion*, edited by James S. Grotstein, 93–102. London: Tavistock Publications.

Jung, Carl Gustav. 1969. *On the Nature of the Psyche*. Translated by Richard F. C. Hull. Princeton, NJ: Princeton University Press.

Kelly, T. 1995. "Holy Saturday." *The Tablet*, April, 15–22.

Kestenberg, Judith. 1956. "On the Development of Maternal Feelings in Early Childhood: Observations and Reflections." *The Psychoanalytic Study of the Child* 11 (1): 257–91.

King James Bible. 2008. *Oxford "Authorized Edition" and the Original (1611) King James version.* Oxford: Oxford University Press.

Kingston, Warren, and Cohen, Jonathan. 1986. "Primal Repression: Clinical and Theoretical Aspects." *International Journal of Psychoanalysis* 67 (3): 337–55.

Klein, Melanie. 1946. "Notes on Some Schizoid Mechanisms." *International Journal of Psychoanalysis* 27: 99–110.

Klein, Sydney. 1981. "Autistic Phenomena in Neurotic Patients." *In Do I Dare Disturb the Universe? A Memorial to Wilfred R. Bion*, edited by James S. Grostein, 103–14. London: Tavistock Publications.

LaMothe, Ryan. 2006. "Constructing Infants: Anthropological Realities and Analytic Horizons." *Psychoanalytic Review* 93 (3): 437–77.

———. 2012. "Potential Space: Creativity, Resistance, and Resiliency in the Face of Racism." *Psychoanalytic Review* 99 (6): 851–76.

Laplanche, Jean, and Jean-Bertrand Pontalis. 1973. *The Language of Psychoanalysis.* Translated by Donald Nicholson-Smith. London and New York: Routledge.

Lemoine-Luccioni, Eugénie. 1987. *The Dividing of Women, Or, Woman's Lot*. Translated by M. Davenport and M. Reguis. London: Free Association Books.

Lewis, Emanuel. 1983. "Stillbirth: Psychological Consequences and Strategies of Management." In *Advances in Perinatal Medicine: Volume 3*, edited by Aubrey

Minsky, Emanuel A. Friedman and Louis Gluck, 205–46. New York: Plenum Publishing.

Lewis, Emanuel, and Stanford Bourne. 1989. "Perinatal Death." *Ballière's Clinical Obstetrics and Gynaecology* 3 (4): 935–53.

Lewis, Emanuel, and Patrick Casement. 1986. "The Inhibitions of Mourning by Pregnancy a Case Study." *Psychoanalytic Psychotherapy* 2 (1): 45–52.

O'Shaughnessy, Edna. 1981. "A Commemorative Essay on W.R. Bion's Theory of Thinking." *Journal of Child Psychotherapy* 7 (2): 181–92.

Mahler, Margaret, Fred Pine, and Anni Bergman. 1975. *The Psychological Birth of the Human Infant: Symbiosis and Individuation.* London: Hutchinson.

Main, Thomas. 1968. "A Fragment on Mothering." In *Psychosocial Nursing: Studies from the Cassel Hospital*, edited by Elizabeth Barnes. London: Tavistock Publications.

Matte-Blanco, Ignacio. 1959. "Expression in Symbolic Logic of the Characteristics of the System UCS or the Logic of the System UCS. *International Journal of Psychoanalysis* 40 (1): 1–5.

———. 1986. "Understanding Matte-Blanco." *International Journal of Psychoanalysis* 67 (2): 251–54.

Mazjels, Neil. 1985. "Self-Envy, the Womb and the Nature of Goodness—A Reappraisal of the Death Instinct." *International Journal of Psychoanalysis* 66 (2): 185–92.

McGinn, Bernard. 1998. *The Flowering of Mysticism: Men and Women in the New Mysticism (1200–1350)*. New York: Crossroad Publishing Company.

Milner, Marion. 1987. *The Suppressed Madness of Sane Men: Forty-four Years of Exploring Psychoanalysis*. Hove and New York: Brunner-Routledge.

Mitchell, Stephen. 1992. *Tao Te Ching: A New English Version*, translated by Stephen Mitchell. New York: HarperCollins.

Nietzsche, Freidrich. 1968. *The Will to Power*, edited by Walter Kaufmann. New York: Vintage Books.

Ogden, Thomas. 1985. "On Potential Space." *International Journal of Psychoanalysis* 66 (2): 129–41.

O'Shane, Pat. "The Psychologigal [*sic*] Impact of White Colonialism on Aboriginal People." *Australasian Psychiatry* 3 (3): 149–53.

O'Shaughnessy, Edna. 1981. "A Commemorative Essay on W.R. Bion's Theory of Thinking." *Journal of Child Psychotherapy* 7 (2): 181–92.

Perry, Bruce, Ronnie Pollard, Toi Blakley, William Baker, and Domenico Vigilante. 1995. "Childhood Trauma, the Neurobiology of Adaptation and Use-Dependent Development of the Brain: How States Become Traits." *Infant Mental Health Journal* 16 (4): 271–91.

Pick, Irma. 1985. "Working Through in the Countertransference." *International Journal of Psychoanalysis* 66 (2): 157–66.

Pines, Dinora. 1972. "Pregnancy and motherhood: interaction between fantasy and reality." *British Journal of Medical Psychology* 45 (4): 333–43.

———. 1982. "The Relevance of Early Psychic Development to Pregnancy and Abortion." *International Journal of Psychoanalysis* 63 (3): 311–19.

———. 1990. "Pregnancy, Miscarriage and Abortion: A Psychoanalytic Perspective." *International Journal of Psychoanalysis* 71 (2): 301–7.

Pontalis, Jean-Bertrand. 1981. *Frontiers in Psychoanalysis: Between the Dream and Physic Pain.* London: Hogarth Press and The Institute of Psychoanalysis.

Rayner, Eric. 1981. "Infinite Experiences, Affects and the Characteristics of the Unconscious." *International Journal of Psychoanalysis* 62 (4): 403–12.

Raphael-Leff, Joan. 1991. *The Psychological Processes of Childbearing*. London: Chapman & Hall.

Schore, Allan. 1994. *Affect Regulation and the Origin of the Self: The Neurobiology of Emotional Development.* Hillsdale, NJ: Lawrence Erlbaum Associates.

———. 1998. "Early Shame Experiences and Infant Brain Development." In Shame: Interpersonal Behavior, Psychopathology, and Culture, edited by Paul Gilbert and Bernice Andrews, 57–77. Oxford: Oxford University Press

Spitz, Rene. 1945. "Hospitalism: An Enquiry into the Genesis of Psychiatric Conditions in Early Childhood." *The Psychoanalytic Study of the Child* 1 (1): 53–75.

Steffens, David, Larry Tupler, K. Krishnan, and R. Ranga. 1993. "The Neurostructural/Neurofunctional Basis of Depression/Mania." *Current Opinion in Psychiatry* 6 (1): 22–26.

Stern, Daniel. 1985. *The Interpersonal World of the Infant: A View from Psychoanalysis and Developmental Psychology*. New York: Basic Books.

———. 1995. *The Motherhood Constellation: A Unified View of Parent-Infant Psychotherapy*. New York: Basic Books.

Tischler, Salo. 1979. "Being with a Psychotic Child: A Psycho-Analytical Approach to the Problems of Parents of Psychotic Children." *International Journal of Psychoanalysis* 60: 29–37.

Tracey, Norma. 1991. "The Psychic Space in Trauma." *Journal of Child Psychotherapy* 17 (2): 29–43.

———. 2000. *Parents of Premature Infants: Their Emotional World.* Whurr Publishers.

———. 2007. "From Oblivion to Being: Faith and Catastrophe." *Psychoanalytic Review* 94 (2): 213–44.

———. 2009. "Precreative Space." *The Psychoanalytic Review* 96 (6): 1025–53.

Tracey, Norma, Peter Blake, Beulah Warren, Helen Hardy, Sylvia Enfield, and Pam Schein. 1995. "A Mother's Narrative of a Premature Birth." *Journal of Child Psychotherapy* 21 (1): 43–64.

Trevarthen, Colwyn. 1980. "The Foundations of Intersubjectivity: Development and Interpersonal and Cooperative Understanding in Infants." In *The Social Foundation of Language and Thought*, edited by David R. Olson. New York: Norton.

———. 1998. "The Concept and Foundations of Infant Intersubjectivity." In Intersubjective Communication and Emotion in Early Ontogeny, edited by Stein Bråten, 15–46. Cambridge: Cambridge University Press.

Tronick, Edward, and Jeffrey Cohn, 1988. "Infant-Mother Face-to-Face Communicative Interaction: Age and Gender Differences in Coordination and the Occurrence of Mis-coordination." *Child Development* 60 (1): 85–92.

Tronick, Edward, Margaret Ricks, and Jeffrey Cohn. 1982. "Maternal and Infant Affective Exchange: Patterns of Adaptive Change." In *Emotion and Early Interaction*, edited by Tiffany Field and Alan Fogel, 83–100. Hillsdale, NJ: Erlbaum.

Tustin, Frances. 1972. *Autism and Childhood Psychosis*. London: Hogarth Press.

———. 1981. "Psychological Birth and Psychological Catastrophe." In *Do I Dare Disturb the Universe? A Memorial to W. R. Bion*, edited by James S. Grotstein, 181–96. Tavistock Publications.

———. 1990a. *The Protective Shell in Children and Adults*. London: Karnac Books.

———. 1990b. "Autistic Encapsulation in Neurotic Patients." In *Master Clinicians on Treating the Regressed Patient*, edited by Bryce Boyer and Peter Giovacchini, 117–38. Northvale, NJ: Jason Aronson.

———. 1994. "Autistic Children Who Are Assessed as not Brain-damaged." *Journal of Child Psychotherapy* 20 (1): 103–31.

Ungunmerr, Miriam-Rose. 1993. "Dadirri: Listening to one another." In *A Spirituality of Catholic Aborigines and the Struggle for Justice*, edited by Joan Hendricks and Gerry Hefferan. Brisbane: Aborigines & Torres Strait Islander Apostolate.

Van der Kolk, Bessel. 1993. "Biological Considerations about Emotions, Trauma, Memory, and the Brain." In *Human Feelings: Explorations in Affect Development and Meaning*, edited by Steven Ablon, Daniel Brown, Edward Khantzian and John Mack, 221–40. Hillsdale, NJ: Analytic Press.

———. 2014. *The Body Keeps the Score: Brian, Mind, and Body in the Healing of Trauma.* New York: Viking Press.

Van der Kolk, Bessel, and Jose Saporta, 1993. "Biological Response to Psychic Trauma." In *International Handbook of Traumatic Stress Syndromes*, edited by John P. Wilson and Beverley Raphael, 25–34. New York: Plenum Press.

Van der Kolk, Bessel, David Pelcovitz, Susan Roth, Francine Mandel, Alexander McFarlane, Judith Herman. 1996. "Dissociation, Somatization, and Affect Regulation: The Complexity of Adaption of Trauma." *American Journal of Psychiatry* 153 (7 Suppl): 83–93.

Williams, Meg Harris. 2010. *The Aesthetic Development: The Poetic Spirit of Psychoanalysis: Essays on Bion, Meltzer, Keats*. London: Karnac Books.

Winnicott, Donald. 1960. "The Theory of the Parent-Infant Relationship." *International Journal of Psychoanalysis*, 41: 585–95.

———. 1965. "Psycho-analysis and the Sense of Guilt [1958]." In *The Maturational Processes and the Facilitating Environment: Studies in the Theory of Emotional Development*, 15–28. London: Karnac Books.

———. 1984a. "Birth Memories, Birth Trauma, and Anxiety [1949]." In *Through Paediatrics to Psychoanalysis: Collected Papers*, 174–193. London and New York: Routledge.

———. 1984b. "Primary maternal preoccupation [1956]." In *Through Paediatrics to Psychoanalysis: Collected Papers*, 300–305. London and New York: Routledge.

———. 1986. "Fear of Breakdown." In *The British School of Psychoanalysis: The Independent Tradition*, edited by Gregorio Kohon. London: Free Association Books.

# Index

# About the Author

Norma Tracey has been a social worker for sixty-three years and a psychoanalytic psychotherapist (NSWIPP) for thirty-one of her forty years of working with mothers and infants. She had a Red Cross Scholarship at Sydney University and worked there for three years before marrying. Returning to work four years later, she was employed as assistant to the Professor of Child Health running seminars, doing home visits with fifth year medical students in the Institute of Child Health, working with mothers and infants with phenylketonuria and coeliac disease, and with patients in the Rheumatic Fever Clinic. She then moved to working in the Department of Child and Family Psychiatry in the same children's hospital, doing intense therapy with parents and children and making marked changes in approaches to infants, child patients and their parents. With Dr. John Yu, she began the first clinical teams for wholistic support of young mothers and their infants. This continues to the present day as a model in that hospital. She also founded the first migrant interpreting service in Australia. She then went into private practice, teaching and supervising in the Institute of Psychoanalytic Psychotherapy for thirty years.

In the last twenty years, she has worked extensively with Aboriginal young mothers and their infants and preschool children. She is the founder of three parent-infant organisations, author or editor of five books, and author of eight booklets and twenty-four internationally published papers. In 2020, she was awarded an Order of Australia for her contribution to mental health in the community and her work with Aboriginal pregnant women and young mothers and their children up to school level. She received the Kath Cleary 2022 Social Justice Award on behalf of the Mercy Foundation for outstanding work and leadership in combining best practice in psychoanalytic therapy with Indigenous Australian spirituality in the Dreaming and Dadirri, making significant contributions to improving the lives of Aboriginal parents, infants and children who have suffered trauma.

# Other Publications by the Author

(Please note my surname was Porteous until 1977)


1. Noonan, K., Porteous, N., Yu J., 1970. "Fantasy Becomes Reality—The Effects of the Birth of a Second Phyleketenuric Infant to a Greek Family." *Australian Journal of Mental Retardation* 1.123.
2. Porteous N., 1971. "Emotional Affects of Celiac Disease on the Mother Child relationship." *Medical Journal Australia.*
3. Hart, J., Porteous, N., 1971. "Mothers Group—An Attempt at Preventative Psychiatry," *Medical Journal Australia*, p. 1405–6.
4. Gardner, A. Porteous N. Walker-Smith, J. A., 1971. "The Emotional affects of Coeliac Disease." *British Paediatric Journal.*
5. Porteous, N., 1973. "What makes a battering Parent?" State Social Work Mental Health Conference. Rozelle Hospital.
6. Porteous, N., 1977. "The Health Care Professional and the Migrant." *Medical Journal Australia*, 1, pp. 891–896
7. Glyer, L., Hayward, T., Tracey, N., Page, C., 1977. "The Family and Mental Retardation." Presented Post Graduate week. RAHC. Published 1990, *NSW Social Work and Genetic Counselling Newsletter*. Vol. 2.
8. Tracey, N., 1990. "The Psychodynamics of Pregnancy." *Australian Journal of Psychotherapy.*
9. Tracey, N., 1991. "The Psychic Space in Trauma." *Journal of Child Psychotherapy London*. Vol. 17, No. 2.
10. Tracey, N., 1993. Mothers and Fathers Speak: On Pregnancy Birth and the First Year of Life. Apollo Press. Australia.
11. Tracey, N., Some Thoughts on Inner-world Processes during Pregnancy. The Child Psychoanalytic Gazette. March 1994.
12. Tracey, N., 1991. Sleep for Mother and Baby.
13. Tracey, N., Blake, P., Warren, B., Hardy, H., Enfield, S., Shein, P., 1995. "A Mothers Narrative of a Premature Birth." Vol. 21, No. 1.

14. Tracey, N., Blake, P., Warren, B., Hardy, H., Enfield, S., Shein, P., 1996. "Will I be to my son as my father was to me." Vol. 22, No. 2, Pp. 168–194.
15. Tracey, N., et al., 2000. "Neonatal Intensive Care: NICU and Infants." *Australian Association for Infant Mental Health Newsletter*.
16. Tracey, N., et al., 2000. "Your Infant and you in Intensive Care." *Welcome Publication.*
17. Tracey, N., "Thinking about and working with depressed mothers in the early months of their infant's life." *Journal of Child Psychotherapy.* London: Routledge. Vol. 26, No. 2, pp.181–205.
18. Tracey, N., 2000. Parents of Premature Infants. London: Whurr Publications.
19. Tracey, N., 2007. "From Oblivion to Being: Faith and Catastrophe." *The Psychoanalytic Review* Vol. 94, No. 2, London. New York.
20. Tracey, N., 2006. "Psychic Space—Aboriginal Dreaming from Spirituality to Violence." Published *The Psychoanalytic Review*. ANZAP Conference.
21. Tracey, N., Australian Dreaming. TRANSGENERATIONALTRAUMA. Presented PPAA Conference 2007.
22. Tracey, N., 2008. "Working in the Preschool Setting—A place to Heal Trans generational Trauma." Aboriginal Preschool Conference. (Keynote Speaker)
23. Tracey, N., 2009. "The Psychic Space in Trauma." *The Psychoanalytic Review* Vol. 96, No. 6, NPAP.
24. Tracey, N., 2010. "Loss of the Dreaming." ANZAP Conference.
25. Tracey, N., 2011, World Congress accepted to present Aboriginal Dreaming and the Autistic Core in trauma.
26. Tracey, N., 2011, World Congress Suicide in Young Aboriginal Men.
27. Tracey, N., 2012, "The Autistic Core in Aboriginal Trauma: Breaking down or Breaking Out of the Autistic Defence." *Psychoanalysis, Culture and Society* Vol. 17, Issue, 4. Special Issue: Psychosis. Guest editor: Marilyn Charles.
28. Tracey, N., 2012. "Working at the interface of education and trauma in an Indigenous preschool." In *Psychodynamic Perspectives on Working with Children, Families, and Schools*, edited by Michael O'Loughlin, pp.133–52 Lanham, MD: Jason Aronson.
29. Tracey, N., 2013. "Psychic space: Aboriginal dreaming from spirituality to violence." *The Psychoanalytic Review.*
30. Tracey, N., 2013. *The Five Big Ideas*. Sydney: Bauer Press and Gunawirra Ltd.

31. Tracey, N., 2013. "Perversion." Paper presented at the New South Wales Institute of Psychoanalytic Psychotherapy (NSWIPP) Conference, Sydney, Australia.
32. Tracey, N., 2013. "The sense of loss and the search for meaning." In *The Ethics of Remembering and the Consequences of Forgetting: Essays on Trauma, History and Memory,* edited by Michael A. O'Loughlin. Lanham, MD: Jason Aronson.
33. Tracey, N., 2015, Thoughts from Michael Eigen in my work with young Aboriginal mothers. In *Living Moments: Tributes to Michael Eigen*, edited by Stephen Bloch and Loray Daws. London: Karnac.
34. Tracey, N., 2016. *Across the Divide*. London: Routledge.
35. Tracey, N., 2016. *Transgenerational Trauma and the Aboriginal Child: Healing through Intervention.* Lanham, MD: Rowman & Littlefield.
36. Hogan, A., Collins, E., Tracey, N., 2022. Nurturing ourselves and our Children. Strong Mothers Booklet.

www.ingramcontent.com/pod-product-compliance
Ingram Content Group UK Ltd.
Pitfield, Milton Keynes, MK11 3LW, UK
UKHW041452071026
15587UKWH00010B/822

9 781666 921267